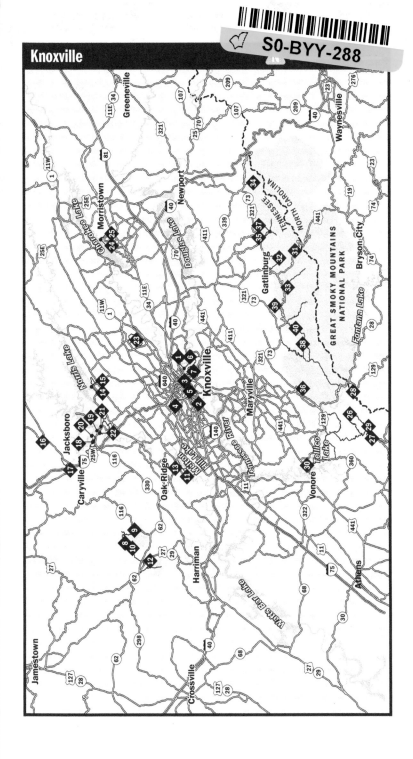

Knoxville

S0-BYY-288

Map Legend

Trailhead

North Indicator

Path Direction

←
Off map
or pinpoint

Capital, Cities
and towns

Interstate highways

U.S. highways

State roads

Other roads

Featured trail

Alternate trail

Boardwalk or stairs

Unpaved roads

State border

County border

Ridgeline

Railroads

River or stream

Water body

STATE PARK
Preserve or
other public land

🏃 Baseball field	■ General point of interest	🏠 Ranger station
⛵ Boat launch	H Hospital	🚻 Restrooms
≍ Bridge	⛏ Mine/quarry	📷 Scenic viewpoint
⛺ Campground	🗿 Monument	◤ Shelter
✝ Cemetery	△ Overlook	🔑 Spring
⛪ Church	P Parking	🏪 Store
🏛 Dam	🏛 Pavilion	🏊 Swimming
🎣 Fishing	▲ Peak	🗼 Tower
⌇ Gate	🎪 Picnic	🏔 Tunnel
		🏞 Waterfall

Overview Map Key

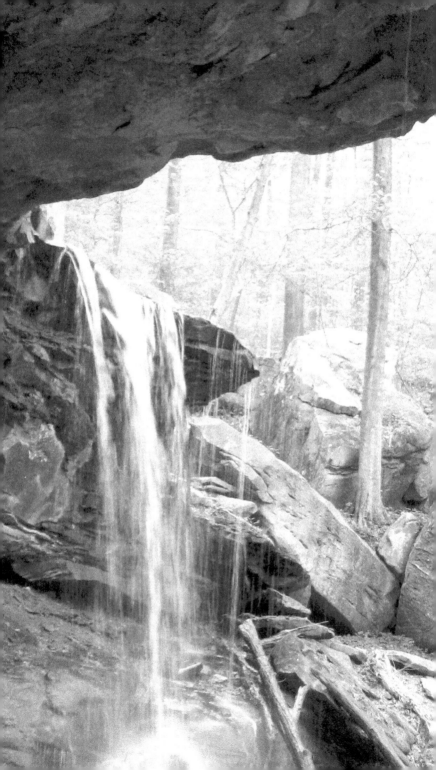

Five-Star Trails

Knoxville

Your Guide to the Area's Most Beautiful Hikes

Johnny Molloy

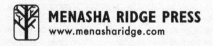
MENASHA RIDGE PRESS
www.menasharidge.com

Five-Star Trails Knoxville
Your Guide to the Area's Most Beautiful Hikes

Copyright © 2011 by Johnny Molloy
All rights reserved
Published by Menasha Ridge Press
Distributed by Publishers Group West
Printed in the United States of America
First edition, first printing

Cover design by Scott McGrew
Text design by Annie Long
Cover photograph by Harold R. Stinnette Photo Stock / Alamy; view of the Smokies
Author photograph by Pam Morgan
All interior photographs by Johnny Molloy
Cartography and elevation profiles by Johnny Molloy, Steve Jones, and
    Scott McGrew

Library of Congress Cataloging-in-Publication Data

Molloy, Johnny, 1961.
Five-star trails, Knoxville : your guide to the area's most beautiful hikes /
Johnny Molloy.
    p. cm. — (Five-star trails)
Summary: "No one knows Knoxville better than veteran outdoor-adventure author
Johnny Molloy. Each hike text displays one- to five-star rankings in five categories:
Scenery, Difficulty, Trail Condition, Solitude, and Appropriateness for Children. Each
entry includes directions to the trailhead, at-a-glance info, a user-friendly map, GPS
coordinates, an elevation profile, and a brief overview"—Provided by publisher.
Includes bibliographical references and index.
ISBN-13: 978-0-89732-922-4 (pbk.); ISBN 978-0-89732-923-1 (ebook)
ISBN-10: 0-89732-922-8 (pbk.); ISBN 978-1-63404-271-0 (hardcover)
1. Hiking—Tennessee—Knoxville—Guidebooks. 2. Trails—Tennessee—
Knoxville—Guidebooks. 3. Knoxville (Tenn.)—Guidebooks. I. Title.
GV199.42.T22K666 2011
917.68'85—dc23
                        2011022117

Menasha Ridge Press
An imprint of AdventureKEEN
2204 First Avenue South, Suite 102
Birmingham, AL 35233
menasharidgepress.com

DISCLAIMER
This book is meant only as a guide to select trails in and near Knoxville, Tennessee.
This book does not guarantee hiker safety in any way—you hike at your own risk.
Neither Menasha Ridge Press nor Johnny Molloy is liable for property loss or
damage, personal injury, or death that result in any way from accessing or hiking the
trails described in the following pages. Please be especially cautious when walking in
potentially hazardous terrains with, for example, steep inclines or drop-offs. Do not
attempt to explore terrain that may be beyond your abilities. Please read carefully the
introduction to this book as well as further safety information from other sources.
Familiarize yourself with current weather reports and maps of the area you plan
to visit (in addition to the maps provided in this guidebook). Be cognizant of park
regulations and always follow them. Do not take chances.

Contents

Dedication

This book is for all of the Tennessee Volunteers.
We are blessed with abundant beauty.

Acknowledgments

Thanks to all of the people who have constructed, maintained, and advocated trails and hiking in Knoxville and East Tennessee. And thanks to all of the people who accompanied me on the trails. My companions include but are not limited to John Cox, Steve "Devo" Grayson, Pam Morgan, Bryan Delay, Karen Stokes, and Tom Lauria.

THE SOUTHERN APPALACHIANS RISE PROUDLY ABOVE KNOXVILLE.

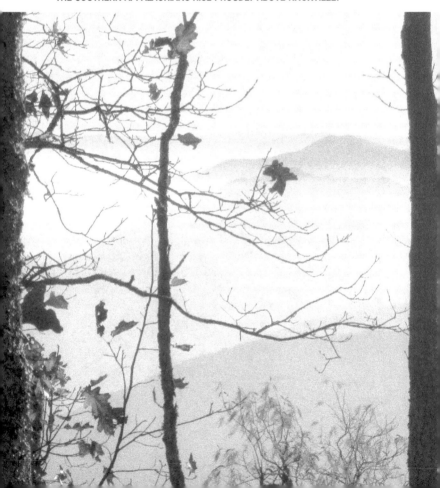

Preface

Knoxville is a hiker's town. People like this sport in higher percentages here than in your average city, that is for certain. If somebody is not an avid hiker, they know someone who is.

Talking about trails in Knoxville is as common as conversation about our beloved Tennessee Volunteers sports programs. Knoxville offers an inordinately large number of stores that cater to the outdoors, far above what you think its population could support. Why is that? The answer is partly geographic and partly cultural.

Geographically speaking, Knoxville couldn't be better situated for terrain and trails on which to trek. The master chain of the Appalachian Range—the Great Smoky Mountains—rises within sight of Knoxville. This span is simply the highest, wildest contiguous plot of rushing streams, rugged ridges, huge trees, colorful wildflowers, and abundant wildlife in the eastern United States. Protected as the Great Smoky Mountains National Park, this area has more than 900 miles of hiking trails within its boundaries. Most of the trailheads on the Tennessee side of the park are within an hour's drive of Knoxville, so residents flock to the Smokies. In fact, if you did a man-on-the-street interview and asked people to say the first thing that came to mind upon hearing the word "hike," the word "Smokies" would likely be chosen most often. So the Smokies sets the stage for hitting the trail and is the backbone of our hiking community in the heart of East Tennessee.

But there are many more places for a trail treader than that magnificent park. The Cumberland Plateau rises to the west of the Tennessee Valley. The Plateau, as it is known in these parts, offers distinctly different terrain with correspondingly unique hiking experiences. Water-carved gorges slice through this elevated table of land, exposing rock walls and creating rock houses, sheer bluffs, and other geological features that complement the green expanse of the Smokies.

And then there is the ridge-and-valley country north of town, a sort of blending of The Plateau and the high ranges to the east. Here, in places like Norris Dam State Park, narrow hollows are flanked by tightly packed ridges (imagine a rumpled carpet), never particularly high, but nonetheless creating an attractive landscape over which to walk.

No flatland itself, the Tennessee Valley embraces the hilly town of Knoxville. And with citizens interested in hiking, it is only natural that trails and greenways aplenty have been created in the greater metropolitan area. They make going out on a walk not only inviting but also convenient.

So hiking in Knoxville can mean a ramble through the wilds of the Great Smokies, a trip to a geological formation on the Cumberland Plateau, a walk in the deep dark hollows of the ridge-and-valley country, or a quick escape on a greenway near your house or lodging. It all depends on your mood, company, and desires. It does not necessarily depend on the weather: You can hike year-round in Knoxville. In the heat of summer, you can escape to the high country, and in the chill of winter, you can still enjoy the trails of the Tennessee River Valley.

The variety of hikes in this book reflects the diversity of this region. Day hikes cover routes of multiple lengths, ranging from easy to difficult. Trail configurations include out-and-backs, loops, balloon loops, and even double loops. Destinations vary from downtown Knoxville to the "back of beyond" in the Smokies. The routes also befit a range of athletic prowess and hiking experience.

Simply scan the table of contents, flip randomly through the book, or utilize the hiking recommendations list on the next page. Find your hike, and get out there and enjoy it. And bring a friend, too. Enjoying nature in the company of another is a great way to enhance your relationship as well as to escape from television, e-mail, Internet, and other electronics that bind us to the daily grind.

—*Johnny Molloy*

Recommended Hikes

Best for Scenery

Best for Wildlife

Best for Seclusion

Best for Kids

Best for Dogs

Best for Water Lovers

Best for Human History

Best for Waterfalls

Best for Geology

Best for Wildflowers

Best for Views

Best for Nature Study

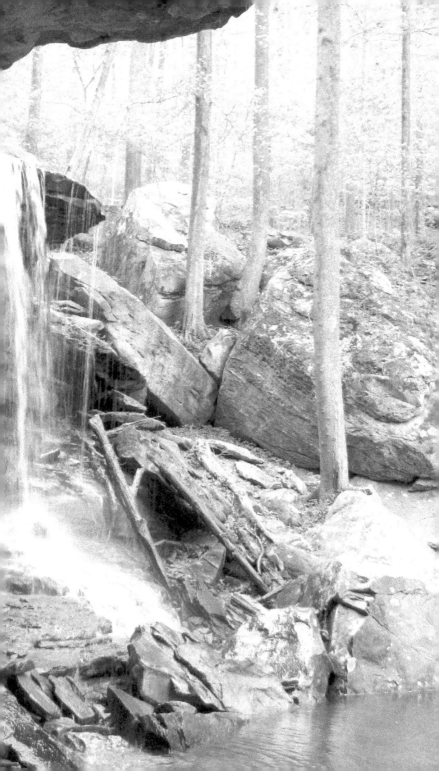

Introduction

About This Book

Five Star Trails: Knoxville details 40 great hikes in this city and its immediate region. Often referred to as the heart of East Tennessee, Knoxville is a great jumping-off point for hikers: it's where immediate urban and suburban trails can satiate scenery-hungry residents, while the superlative beauty of the adjacent national and state parks is just a short drive away. All this adds up to a hiker's nirvana.

Greater Knoxville's Geographic Divisions

The hikes in this book have been divided into five geographic regions. Altogether, they embrace great destinations such as urban greenways, Great Smoky Mountains National Park, Cherokee National Forest, the Cumberland Plateau, Big Ridge State Park, Panther Creek State Park, Fort Loudon State Park, and much more.

* **KNOXVILLE** covers the city core. The hikes here follow mainly along Knoxville's abundant and expanding greenway system. Choose them for a quick escape for daily exercise or to explore nature parks such as Ijams or William Hastie Natural Area.

* **WEST** encompasses the city of Oak Ridge and public lands west of town, including the Cumberland Plateau. Hike along interpretive trails at the Oak Ridge Arboretum or climb to the highest point on the Cumberland Plateau at Frozen Head State Park. Or try a lakeside greenway.

* **NORTH** takes in the ridge-and-valley country north of Knoxville and the northward part of the Cumberland Plateau. In this area, you can hike trails around Norris Dam, with views aplenty and wildflowers galore, or take a geologically rewarding trek on the Cumberland Trail, Tennessee's master path.

* **EAST** stretches from House Mountain State Natural Area to Panther Creek State Park. House Mountain is the highest point in Knox County and has views rivaling the Smokies. Panther Creek State

WATERFALLS CAN BE FOUND IN ALL DIRECTIONS FROM KNOXVILLE.

Park is unheralded as a hiking destination. The varied topography and combination of land and water will leave you wondering why you haven't been there before.

★ **SOUTH** includes the highest terrain in the region, from the incomparable Smoky Mountains to the remote and unrefined Cherokee National Forest. The Smokies destinations in this guidebook lie within an easy drive from Knoxville and include a park medley of pioneer homesteads, panoramic overlooks, and intense waterfalls. The Cherokee trails offer scenery and destinations comparable to the Smokies, minus the crowds, and these routes add a primitive component lacking in the Smokies' more developed pathways.

The trail-laced geographic regions of greater Knoxville create a mosaic of natural splendor that will please even the most discriminating hiker.

How to Use This Guidebook

The following information walks you through this guidebook's organization to make it easy and convenient for you to plan great hikes.

OVERVIEW MAP, MAP KEY, & MAP LEGEND

The overview map on the inside front cover depicts the location of the primary trailhead for all 40 of the hikes described in this book. The numbers shown on the overview map pair with the map key on the opposite page. Each hike's number remains with that hike throughout the book. Thus, if you spot an appealing hiking area on the overview map, you can flip through the book and find those hikes easily by their numbers at the top of each profile page.

TRAIL MAPS

In addition to the overview map, a detailed map of each hike's route appears with its profile. On each of these maps, symbols indicate the trailhead, the complete route, significant features, facilities, and topographic landmarks such as creeks, overlooks, and peaks. A legend identifying the map symbols used throughout the book appears on the inside back cover.

To produce the highly accurate maps in this book, I used a handheld GPS unit to gather data while hiking each route, and then sent that data to the publisher's expert cartographers.

Further, despite the high quality of the maps in this guidebook, the publisher and I strongly recommend that you always carry an additional map, such as the ones noted in each hike profile's introductory listing for "Maps."

ELEVATION PROFILE (DIAGRAM)

This diagram represents the rises and falls of the trail as viewed from the side, over the complete distance (in miles) of that trail. On the diagram's vertical axis, or height scale, the number of feet indicated between each tick mark lets you visualize the climb. To avoid making flat hikes look steep and steep hikes appear flat, varying height scales provide an accurate image of each hike's climbing difficulty. For example, one hike's scale might rise to 2,000 feet, while another goes to 4,800 feet.

Also, each entry will list the elevation at the hike *trailhead* as well as the elevation *peak* if there is any notable elevation change for that trail. Otherwise, the entry will indicate simply the trailhead elevation.

THE HIKE PROFILE

This book contains a concise and informative narrative of each hike from beginning to end. The text will get you from a well-known road or highway to the trailhead, to the twists and turns of the hike route, back to the trailhead, and to notable nearby attractions, if there are any. Each profile opens with the route's star ratings, GPS trailhead coordinates, and other key information. Below is an explanation of the introductory elements that give you a snapshot of each of this book's 40 routes.

STAR RATINGS

Five-Star Trails is the Menasha Ridge Press series of guidebooks geared to specific cities across the United States, such as this one for

Knoxville. Following is the explanation for the rating system of one to five stars in each of the five categories.

FOR SCENERY:

★ ★ ★ ★ ★   Unique, picturesque panoramas

★ ★ ★ ★   Diverse vistas

★ ★ ★   Pleasant views

★ ★   Unchanging landscape

★   Not selected for scenery

FOR TRAIL CONDITION:

★ ★ ★ ★ ★   Consistently well maintained

★ ★ ★ ★   Stable, with no surprises

★ ★ ★   Average terrain to negotiate

★ ★   Inconsistent, with good and poor areas

★   Rocky, overgrown, or often muddy

FOR CHILDREN:

★ ★ ★ ★ ★   Babies in strollers are welcome

★ ★ ★ ★   Fun for anyone past the toddler stage

★ ★ ★   Good for young hikers with proven stamina

★ ★   Not enjoyable for children

★   Not advisable for children

FOR DIFFICULTY:

★ ★ ★ ★ ★   Grueling

★ ★ ★ ★   Strenuous

★ ★ ★   Moderate (won't beat you up—but you'll know you've been hiking)

★ ★   Easy with patches of moderate

★   Good for a relaxing stroll

FOR SOLITUDE:

★ ★ ★ ★ ★   Positively tranquil

★ ★ ★ ★   Spurts of isolation

★ ★ ★   Moderately secluded

★ ★   Crowded on weekends and holidays

★   Steady stream of individuals and/or groups

GPS TRAILHEAD COORDINATES

As noted in "Trail Maps," on pages 2–3, I used a handheld GPS unit to obtain geographic data and sent the information to the publisher's cartographers. In the opener for each hike profile, I have provided the intersection of the latitude (north) and longitude (west) coordinates to orient you at the trailhead. In some cases, you can drive within viewing distance of a trailhead. Other hikes require a short walk to reach the trailhead from a parking area. Either way, the trailhead coordinates are given from the trail's actual head—its point of origin.

You will also note that this guidebook uses the degree–decimal minute format for presenting the GPS coordinates.

The latitude and longitude grid system is likely quite familiar to you, but here is a refresher, pertinent to visualizing the GPS coordinates: imaginary lines of latitude—called parallels and situated approximately 69 miles apart—run horizontally around the globe. Each parallel is indicated by degrees from the equator (established to be 0°): up to 90°N at the North Pole and down to 90°S at the South Pole.

Imaginary lines of longitude—called meridians—run perpendicular to latitude lines. Longitude lines are likewise indicated by degrees: starting from 0° at the Prime Meridian in Greenwich, England, they continue to the east and west until they meet 180° later at the International Date Line in the Pacific Ocean. At the equator, longitude lines also are approximately 69 miles apart, but that distance narrows as the meridians converge toward the North and South poles.

To convert GPS coordinates given in degrees, minutes, and seconds to the format shown above in degrees–decimal minutes, the seconds are divided by 60. For more on GPS technology, visit **usgs.gov.**

DISTANCE & CONFIGURATION

The distance shown is for the hike from start to finish, as recorded with the GPS unit. There may be options to shorten or extend the hike, but the mileage corresponds to the hike described. The configuration defines the trail as a loop, an out-and-back (taking you in and out via the same route), a figure-eight, or a balloon. As the mileage is for the total hike, it is measured round-trip.

HIKING TIME

Unlike distance, which is a real, measured number, hiking time is an estimate. Every hiker has a different pace. In this guidebook, you can assume the hiking time is based on a pace of about 2 miles per hour (when taking notes and pictures), and that is the standard for most of the hike times. There are some adjustments for steepness, rough terrain, and high elevation. And there is some time built in for a quick breather here and there, but hikers should consider that any prolonged break (such as lunch or swimming) will add to the hike time.

HIGHLIGHTS

Waterfalls, historic sites, or other features that draw hikers to the trail are capsuled here.

ELEVATION

In each trail's opener, you will see the elevation at the trailhead and another figure for the peak height on that route. The full hike profile will also include a complete elevation profile (see above).

ACCESS

Fees or permits required to hike the trail are indicated here, and it is noted if there are none. Trail-access hours are also listed here.

MAPS

This section recommends map sources in addition to the maps in this guidebook.

FACILITIES

For planning your hike, it's helpful to know what to expect at the trailhead or nearby in terms of restrooms, phones, water, and other niceties.

WHEELCHAIR ACCESS

For each hike, you will see its feasibility for outdoor enthusiasts who use a wheelchair.

COMMENTS

Here you will find assorted nuggets of information, such as whether or not your dog is allowed on the trails.

CONTACTS

You'll find phone numbers and websites here for checking trail conditions and gleaning other day-to-day information.

Overview, Route Details, Nearby Attractions, & Directions

Each profile contains a complete narrative of the hike: "Overview" gives you a quick summary of what to expect on that trail. "Route Details" guides you on the hike, start to finish. "Nearby Attractions" suggests other area sites that you might like, such as restaurants, museums, or other trails. "Directions" will get you to the trailhead from a well-known road or highway.

Weather

Each of the four seasons lays its distinct hands on Knoxville. Summer can be fairly hot, but that is when hikers head for the mountains. If you're hiking in Knoxville during summer, I recommend going early in the morning or late in the evening, as thunderstorms can pop up in the afternoons.

Hikers really hit the trails when fall's first northerly fronts sweep cool, clear air across East Tennessee. Mountaintop vistas are best enjoyed during this time. Fall is the driest of all seasons here, and crisp mornings give way to warm afternoons.

Winter can bring frigid subfreezing days and chilling rains—and snow in the high country. However, a brisk hiking pace will keep you warm. Each cold month has several days of mild weather.

Spring will be even more variable. A warm day can be followed by a cold one. Extensive spring rains bring regrowth, but also keep hikers indoors. Still, any avid trekker will find more good hiking days than they will have time to take on in spring and every other season.

The chart below details Knoxville's monthly averages to give you an idea of what weather to expect. (Note: Expect cooler temperatures on the Cumberland Plateau and in the Smokies.)

MONTHLY WEATHER AVERAGES FOR KNOXVILLE, TN			
MONTH	HI TEMP	LO TEMP	RAIN
January	47°F	30°F	4.79"
February	52°F	33°F	3.91"
March	61°F	40°F	5.04"
April	71°F	48°F	3.52"
May	78°F	57°F	4.33"
June	85°F	65°F	4.77"
July	88°F	69°F	3.97"
August	87°F	68°F	3.40"
September	81°F	62°F	3.03"
October	71°F	52°F	3.03"
November	60°F	41°F	4.10"
December	50°F	34°F	4.37"

Water

How much is enough? Well, one simple physiological fact should convince you to err on the side of excess when deciding how much water to pack: a hiker walking steadily in 90° heat needs approximately 10 quarts of fluid per day. That's 2.5 gallons. A good rule of thumb is to hydrate prior to your hike, carry (and drink) 6 ounces of water for every mile you plan to hike, and hydrate again after the hike. For most people, the pleasures of hiking make carrying water a relatively minor price to pay to remain safe and healthy. So pack more water than you anticipate needing even for short hikes.

If you are tempted to drink "found water," do so with extreme caution. Many ponds and lakes encountered by hikers are fairly stagnant and their water tastes terrible. Drinking such water presents inherent risks for thirsty trekkers. *Giardia* parasites contaminate many water sources and cause the dreaded intestinal giardiasis that can last for weeks after ingestion. For information, visit The Centers for Disease Control website at cdc.gov/parasites/giardia.

In any case, effective treatment is essential before using any water source found along the trail. Boiling water for 2 to 3 minutes is always a safe measure for camping, but day hikers can consider iodine tablets, approved chemical mixes, filtration units rated for *Giardia*, and UV filtration. Some of these methods (e.g., filtration with an added carbon filter) remove bad tastes typical in stagnant water, while others add their own taste. As a precaution, carry a means of water purification in case you underestimate your consumption needs.

Clothing

Weather, unexpected trail conditions, fatigue, extended hiking duration, and wrong turns can individually or collectively turn a great outing into a very uncomfortable one at best—and a life-threatening one at worst. Thus, proper attire plays a key role in staying comfortable and, sometimes, staying alive. Below are some helpful guidelines.

★ Choose silk, wool, or synthetics for maximum comfort in all of your hiking attire—from hats to socks and in between. Cotton is fine if the weather remains dry and stable, but you won't be happy if it gets wet.

★ Always wear a hat, or at least tuck one into your day pack or hitch it to your belt. Hats offer all-weather sun and wind protection as well as warmth if it turns cold.

★ Be ready to layer up or down as the day progresses and the mercury rises or falls. Today's outdoor wear makes layering easy, with such designs as jackets that convert to vests and zip-off or button-up legs.

★ Wear hiking boots or sturdy hiking sandals with toe protection. Flip-flopping on a paved path in an urban botanical garden is one thing, but never hike a trail in open sandals or casual sneakers. Your bones and arches need support, and your skin needs protection.

★ Pair that footwear with good socks! If you prefer not to sheathe your feet when wearing hiking sandals, tuck the socks into your day pack; you may need them if the weather plummets or if you hit rocky turf and pebbles begin to irritate your feet. And, in an emergency, if you have lost your gloves, you can adapt the socks into mittens.

★ Don't leave rainwear behind, even if the day dawns clear and sunny. Tuck into your day pack, or tie around your waist, a jacket that is breathable and either water-resistant or waterproof. Investigate different choices at your local outdoors retailer. If you are a frequent hiker, ideally you'll have more than one rainwear weight, material, and style in your closet to protect you in all seasons in your regional climate and hiking microclimates.

Essential Gear

Today you can buy outdoor vests that have up to 20 pockets shaped and sized to carry everything from toothpicks to binoculars or, if you don't aspire to feel like a burro, you can neatly stow all of these items in your day pack or backpack. The following list showcases never-hike-without-them items.

★ Water (As emphasized more than once in this book, bring more than you think you will drink; depending on your destination, you may want to bring a water bottle and iodine or filter for purifying water in the wilderness in case you run out.)

★ Map(s) and high-quality compass (Even if you know the terrain from previous hikes, don't leave home without these tools. If you are versed in GPS usage, bring that device, too, but don't rely on it as your sole navigational tool, as batteries can die.)

★ A pocketknife and/or multitool

★ Flashlight or headlamp with extra bulb and batteries

★ Windproof matches and/or a lighter, as well as a fire starter

★ Extra food (trail mix, granola bars, or other high-energy foods)

★ Extra clothes (raingear, warm hat, gloves, and change of socks and shirt)

★ Whistle (This little gadget will be your best friend in an emergency.)

★ Insect repellent

★ Sunscreen (Note the expiration date on the tube or bottle; it's usually embossed on the top.)

First-aid Kit

In addition to the items listed under "Essential Gear," those below may appear overwhelming for a day hike. But any paramedic will tell you that the products listed here, in alphabetical order, are just the basics. The reality of hiking is that you can be out for a week of backpacking and acquire only a mosquito bite, or you can hike for an hour, slip, and suffer a bleeding abrasion or broken bone. Fortunately, these items will collapse into a very small space, and convenient, prepackaged kits are available at your pharmacy and on the Internet.

★ Ace bandages or Spenco joint wraps

★ Ointment (Neosporin or the generic equivalent)

★ Athletic tape

★ Band-Aids

★ Benadryl or the generic equivalent diphenhydramine (in case of allergic reactions)

★ Blister kit (such as Moleskin/Spenco Second Skin)

★ Butterfly-closure bandages

★ Epinephrine in a prefilled syringe (usually by prescription only, and for people known to have severe allergic reactions to such things as bee stings)

★ Gauze (one roll and a half-dozen 4-x-4-inch pads)

★ Hydrogen peroxide or iodine

★ Ibuprofen or acetaminophen

Note: Please consider your intended terrain and the number of hikers in your party before you exclude any article cited above. A botanical garden stroll may not inspire you to carry a complete kit, but anything beyond that warrants precaution. When hiking alone, you should always be prepared for a medical need. And if you are a twosome or with a group, one or more people in your party should be equipped with first-aid material.

General Safety

The following tips may have the familiar ring of your mother's voice as you take note of them.

★ *Always let someone know where you will be hiking and how long you expect to be gone.* It's a good idea to give that person a copy of your route, particularly if you are headed into any isolated area. Let them know when you return.

★ *Always sign in and out of any trail registers provided.* Don't hesitate to comment on the trail condition if space is provided; that's your opportunity to alert others to any problems you encounter.

★ *Do not count on a cell phone for your safety.* Reception may be spotty or nonexistent on the trail, even on an urban walk—especially if it is embraced by towering trees.

★ *Always carry food and water,* even for a short hike.

★ *Ask questions.* State forest and park employees are there to help. It's a lot easier to ask advice beforehand, and it will help you avoid a mishap away from civilization when it's too late to amend an error.

★ *Stay on designated trails.* Even on the most clearly marked trails, there is usually a point where you have to stop and consider in which direction to head. If you become disoriented, don't panic. As soon as you think you may be off track, stop, assess your current direction, and then retrace your steps to the point where you went astray. Using a map, a compass, GPS, and this book, and keeping in mind what you have passed thus far, reorient yourself, and trust your judgment on which way to continue. If you become absolutely unsure of how to continue, return to your vehicle the way you came in. Should you become completely lost and have no idea how to return to the trailhead, remaining in place along the trail and waiting for help is most often the best option for adults and always the best option for children.

★ *Always carry a whistle.* It may be a lifesaver (or at least a major stress reducer) if you do become lost or sustain an injury.

★ *Be especially careful when crossing streams.* Whether you are fording the stream or crossing on a log, make every step count. If you have any doubt about maintaining your balance on a log, ford the stream instead: use a trekking pole or stout stick for balance and face upstream as you cross. If a stream seems too deep to ford, turn back. Whatever is on the other side is not worth risking your life.

★ *Be careful at overlooks.* While these areas may provide spectacular views, they are potentially hazardous. Stay back from the edge of outcrops and be absolutely sure of your footing; a misstep can mean a nasty and possibly fatal fall.

★ *Standing dead trees and storm-damaged living trees pose a real hazard to hikers.* These trees may have loose or broken limbs that could fall at any time. While walking beneath trees, and when choosing a spot to rest or enjoy your snack, look up!

★ *Know the symptoms of hypothermia.* Shivering and forgetfulness are the two most common indicators of this stealthy killer. Hypothermia can occur at any elevation, even in the summer, especially when the hiker is wearing lightweight cotton clothing. If symptoms present themselves, get to shelter, hot liquids, and dry clothes ASAP.

★ *Most important of all, take along your brain.* A cool, calculating mind is the single most important asset on the trail. Think before you act. Watch your step. Plan ahead. Avoiding accidents before they happen is the best way to ensure a rewarding and relaxing hike.

Watchwords for Flora & Fauna

BLACK BEARS: Though attacks by black bears are very rare, they have happened in East Tennessee. The sight or approach of a bear can give anyone a start. If you encounter a bear while hiking, remain calm and never run away. Make loud noises to scare off the bear and back away slowly. In primitive and remote areas, assume bears are present; in more developed sites, check on the current bear situation prior to hiking. Most encounters are food related, as bears have an exceptional sense of smell and not particularly discriminating tastes. While this is of greater concern to backpackers and campers, on a day hike, you may plan a lunchtime picnic or will munch on a power bar or other snack from time to time. So remain aware and alert.

MOSQUITOES: These little naggers are more often found in Knoxville but sparingly in the hillier Plateau and Southern

Appalachians. Insect repellent and/or repellent-impregnated clothing are the only simple methods to ward off these pests. In some areas, mosquitoes are known to carry the West Nile virus, so all due caution should be taken to avoid their bites.

POISON IVY, OAK, AND SUMAC: Recognizing and avoiding poison ivy, oak, and sumac are the most effective ways to prevent the painful, itchy rashes associated with these plants. Poison ivy occurs as a vine or groundcover, 3 leaflets to a leaf; poison oak occurs as either a vine or shrub, also with 3 leaflets; and poison sumac flourishes in swampland, each leaf having 7 to 13 leaflets.

Urushiol, the oil in the sap of these plants, is responsible for the rash. Within 14 hours of exposure, raised lines and/or blisters will appear on the affected area, accompanied by a terrible itch. Refrain from scratching; bacteria under your fingernails can cause an infection. Wash and dry the affected area thoroughly, applying a calamine lotion to help dry out the rash. If itching or blistering is severe, seek medical attention. If you do come into contact with one of these plants, remember that oil-contaminated clothes, pets, or hiking gear can easily cause an irritating rash on you or someone else, so wash not only any exposed parts of your body but also clothes, gear, and pets if applicable.

SNAKES: Rattlesnakes, cottonmouths, copperheads, and corals are among the most common venomous snakes in the United States, and hibernation season is typically October through April. In East Tennessee, you will possibly encounter the timber rattler or copperhead. However, the snakes you most likely will see while hiking will be nonvenomous species and subspecies. The best rule is to leave all snakes alone, give them a wide berth as you hike past, and make sure any hiking companions (including dogs) do the same.

When hiking, stick to well-used trails and wear over-the-ankle boots and loose-fitting long pants. Rattlesnakes like to bask in the sun and won't bite unless threatened. Do not step or put your hands beyond where you can clearly see, and avoid wandering around in the dark. Step *onto* logs and rocks, never *over* them, and be especially careful when climbing rocks. Always avoid walking through dense brush or willow thickets. Copperheads are most often found along streams or on a sunny spot atop a rock.

TICKS: Ticks are often found on brush and tall grass, where they seem to be waiting to hitch a ride on a warm-blooded passerby. Adult ticks are most active April into May and again October into November. Among the varieties of ticks, the black-legged tick, commonly called the deer tick, is the primary carrier of Lyme disease. Wear light-colored clothing so ticks can be spotted before they make it to the skin. And be sure to visually check your hair, the back of your neck, armpits, and socks at the end of the hike. During your post-hike shower, take a moment to do a more complete body check. For ticks that are already embedded, removal with tweezers is best. Use disinfectant solution on the wound.

HUNTING: Separate rules, regulations, and licenses govern the various hunting types and related seasons. Though there are generally no problems, hikers may wish to forgo their trips during the big-game seasons, usually in November and December, when the woods suddenly seem filled with orange and camouflage. In East Tennessee, the places you may encounter hunters will be the Cherokee National Forest and some wildlife management areas through which hiking trails travel.

Trail Etiquette

Always treat the trail, wildlife, and fellow hikers with respect. Here are some reminders.

★ Plan ahead in order to be self-sufficient at all times; for example, carry necessary supplies for changes in weather or other conditions. A well-executed trip is a satisfaction to you and to others.

★ Hike on open trails only.

★ Respect trail and road closures (ask if not sure), avoid possible trespassing on private land, and obtain all permits and authorization as required. Also, leave gates as you found them or as marked.

★ Be courteous to other hikers, bikers, equestrians, and others you encounter on the trails.

★ Never spook animals. An unannounced approach, a sudden movement, or a loud noise startles most animals. A surprised animal can be dangerous to you, to others, and to itself. Give them plenty of space.

★ Observe the yield signs that are displayed around the region's trailheads and backcountry. They advise hikers to yield to horses, and bikers to yield to both horses and hikers. A common courtesy on hills is that hikers and bikers yield to any uphill traffic. When encountering mounted riders or horse packers, hikers can courteously step off the trail, on the downhill side if possible. Speak to the riders before they reach you and do not dart behind trees. You are less spooky if the horse can see and hear you. Resist the urge to pet horses unless you are invited to do so.

★ Leave only footprints. Be sensitive to the ground beneath you. This also means staying on the existing trail and not blazing any new trails.

★ Be sure to pack out what you pack in. No one likes to see the trash someone else has left behind.

Tips on Enjoying Hiking in Greater Knoxville

Before you go, read the hike descriptions in this book. Note the website address and phone number in the opener for each trail route, visit the website of the intended hiking destination, and call ahead if you have unanswered questions.

Investigate different areas of East Tennessee. The Smokies is the hiking kingpin, no doubt, but expand your horizons literally with a trip to the Cumberland Plateau, or check out a local greenway. Try new places. Take a chance and make a new adventure instead of trying to re-create the same one over and over. You'll be pleasantly surprised to see so many distinct landscapes in greater Knoxville.

Take your time along the trails. Pace yourself. Our area is filled with wonders both big and small. Don't rush past a tiny salamander to get to that overlook. Stop and smell the wildflowers. Go ahead and take a seat on a trailside rock. Peer into a stream to find secretive fish. Take pictures. Make memories. Don't miss the trees for the forest.

We can't always schedule our free time when we want, but try to hike during the week and avoid the traditional holidays if possible. Trails that are packed in the summer are often clear during the colder months. If you are hiking on a busy day, go early in the morning to enhance your chances of seeing wildlife. The trails really clear out during rainy times, which you might consider for your outing; however, don't hike during a thunderstorm.

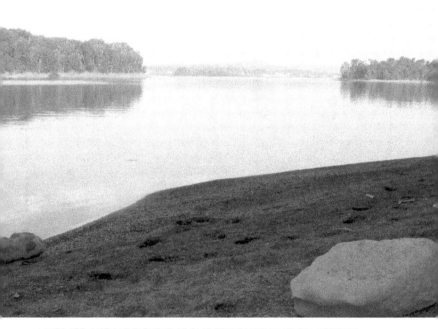

LAKES ARE JUST ONE ELEMENT OF EAST TENNESSEE'S NATURAL HERITAGE.

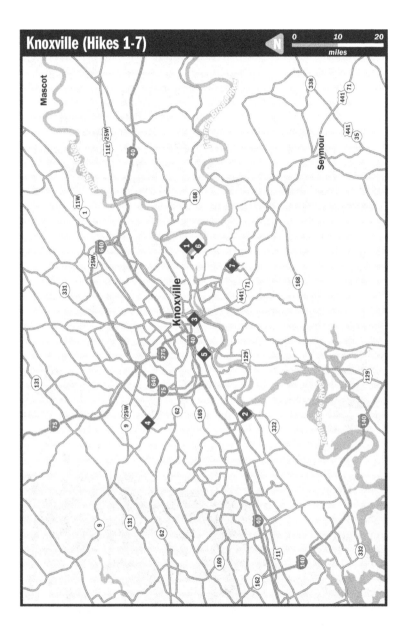

Knoxville

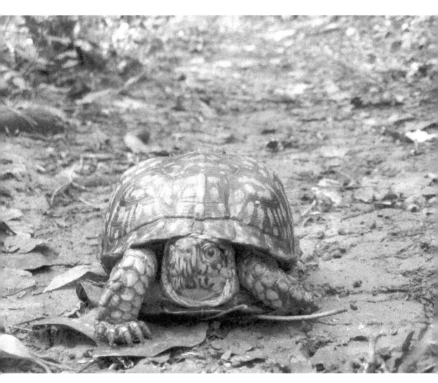

EVEN THE TURTLES LIKE KNOXVILLE'S TRAILS.

Ijams Nature Center Loop

SCENERY: ★ ★ ★
TRAIL CONDITION: ★ ★ ★ ★
CHILDREN: ★ ★ ★ ★
DIFFICULTY: ★ ★
SOLITUDE: ★

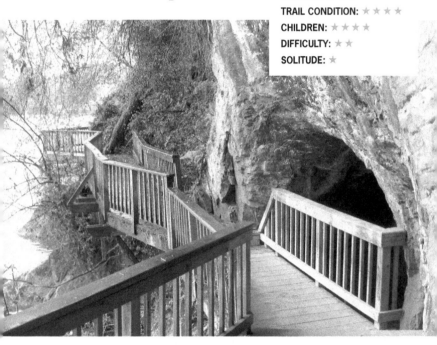

ENJOY THE BOARDWALK THAT SQUEEZES BETWEEN A BLUFF AND THE TENNESSEE RIVER.

GPS TRAILHEAD COORDINATES: N35° 57.335' W83° 52.096'

DISTANCE & CONFIGURATION: 3-mile double loop with spurs

HIKING TIME: 1.8 hours

HIGHLIGHTS: Environmental education, river views, history

ELEVATION: 835 feet at low point to 1,160 feet at high point

ACCESS: No fees, permits, or passes required; open dawn to dusk

MAPS: Ijams Nature Center Trails, USGS Shooks Gap

FACILITIES: Restrooms, water fountain at Ijams Visitor Center

WHEELCHAIR ACCESS: Yes, on nearby Universal Trail

COMMENTS: Other nature trails are available.

CONTACTS: Knoxville Parks and Recreation–Ijams Nature Center, 2915 Island Home Ave., Knoxville, TN 37920; (865) 215-4311; **ci.knoxville.tn.us/parks**

Overview

This hike uses a series of trails to make a pair of loops at Ijams. Leave the worth-a-visit visitor center and raptor enclosure and bisect wooded hills to reach Mead's Quarry. Here, you circle around the lake left over after marble mining operations ceased. The circuit makes a big climb above the quarry, reaching a pair of overlooks. It then heads toward the Tennessee River, making a side trip to Toll Creek, then explores a bluff-side boardwalk over the river. See Maude Moore's Cave; pass by a wildflower-rich hillside near Otter Island, then climb back to the nature center.

Route Details

Now in its fifth decade, Ijams Nature Center continues to be a popular destination for Knoxville residents. Originally the home and property of Alice Ijams in the early 1900s, the grounds were opened to the public in 1965 by the city of Knoxville. Through the years the park has expanded in size, environmental education opportunities, and trail mileage. Today, the nature center utilizes 160 acres to display and protect this urban green space. On this hike you will cover most of the park grounds. On return visits, you can make hiking loops of your own, altering routes to accommodate your companions. The spring wildflowers are one reason to visit, but any time of year you will find something worth seeing.

Facing the visitor center with your back to a nearby pavilion, head right, easterly, to pass under a covered trailhead. Walk left a few feet, then turn right on South Cove Trail, a mulched path. Shortly, pass the Tower Trail on your left, then the Beech Trail on your right, while hiking beneath a second-growth hardwood forest. Descend to reach the wide River Trail at 0.3 miles. Turn right here, toward Mead's Quarry, briefly joining the Will Skelton Greenway, also detailed in this guidebook (see page 46).

Travel south on the asphalt greenway for a short distance, then turn right to carefully cross Island Home Avenue, entering the Mead's

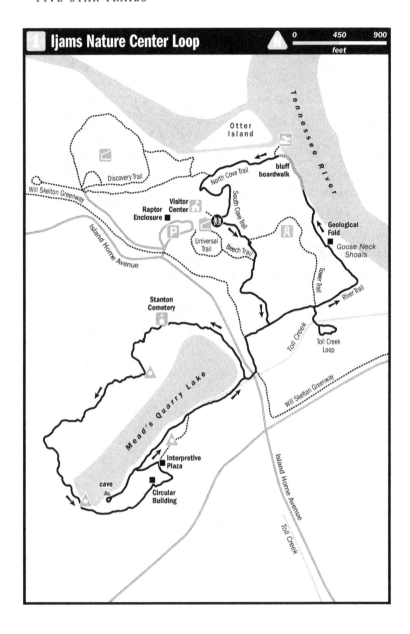

Ijams Nature Center Loop

0   450   900
feet

Tennessee River

Otter Island

bluff boardwalk

North Cove Trail

Discovery Trail

Will Skelton Greenway

South Cove Trail

Raptor Enclosure

Visitor Center

Geological Fold

Goose Neck Shoals

Universal Trail

Beech Trail

Island Home Avenue

Tower Trail

River Trail

Stanton Cemetery

Toll Creek Loop

Toll Creek

Mead's Quarry Lake

Will Skelton Greenway

Interpretive Plaza

cave

Circular Building

Island Home Avenue

Toll Creek

Quarry site. This area was mined for pink marble, used in buildings throughout the United States, from the 1890s to the 1970s. Water naturally filled the quarry after it was dug out, leaving an attractive lake backed by tall granite bluffs.

This hike picks up Tharpe Trace, curving around the right side of the lake. Briefly follow an old road, then veer right onto a dirt path, climbing to reach Stanton Cemetery. Note the marked and unmarked graves, with some of the tombstones hand-inscribed. Many of those interred actually worked at Mead's Quarry.

Less energetic hikers may skip this loop, but for a beautiful vista, continue climbing beyond the cemetery to an overlook at 0.8 miles. Look down on the blue water and scan the surrounding hills and homes beyond the nature center. Reach a high point of 1,160 feet at 1 mile. You just climbed 330 feet from Island Home Avenue.

The downgrade eases at 1.2 miles, where another overlook allows a long view of the lake below. Look for old brick, cut block, and cables—all relics from when this quarry was in operation. Pass a spur trail to a circular structure that is painted to resemble a bird. Proceed to a flat area known as the Interpretive Plaza and reach a trail junction at 1.4 miles. An alluring lake overlook and picnic shelter stand to the right, but this hike goes left, southwesterly on Pink Marble Trace.

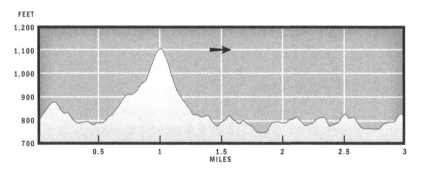

Shortly, you'll reach 25-acre Mead's Quarry Lake. Stay left, heading for Mead's Quarry Cave, which features a stream flowing into Mead's Quarry Lake. Stairs and a boardwalk allow you to peer inside the home of endangered cave species such as bats and salamanders. Pink Marble Trace travels along the water, passing aquatic access paths. This part of the hike demonstrates how to turn an eyesore into an eye pleaser. What once was an abandoned quarry is now the centerpiece of a trail network. Leave the quarry site and return to Island Home Avenue at 1.9 miles.

The Will Skelton Greenway, just across the road, takes you back to the River Trail. Keep northeasterly on the River Trail and make a four-way junction at 2.1 miles. Take the Toll Creek Loop as it drops to a boardwalk, crossing Toll Creek twice. The urban stream has its beauty—and garbage, strewn by litterbugs and then washed into the creek. Now take the River Trail to the Tennessee River, passing a stairway leading up to an interesting geological formation—folded rock strata with the layers easily visible. At 2.5 miles, join my favorite highlight: a bluff boardwalk overhanging the Tennessee River. Take it to work your way around the steep bluff. River views are extensive. Peer into Maude Moore's Cave, with its two entrances now barred.

Curve away from the Tennessee, passing a spur to a boat dock, where boaters can access the nature center. Come near Otter Island, then reach a trail junction at 2.8 miles. Stay left with the North Cove Trail, ascending on a wildflower-covered hill. Come behind the nature center and then complete your loop at 3 miles.

Nearby Attractions

Other hiking opportunities branch out from the Ijams trailhead. From the Ijams entrance, the Will Skelton Greenway extends westerly 1.2 miles to Island Home Park.

Directions

From the intersection of Cumberland Avenue and Gay Street in downtown Knoxville, drive south over the Tennessee River on the Gay Street Bridge to reach a traffic light. Keep forward at the light, now on Sevier Avenue. Travel Sevier Avenue for 0.6 miles, then stay left on Island Home Avenue as Sevier Avenue curves right over railroad tracks. Stay on Island Home Avenue for 2 miles to reach Ijams Nature Center on your left.

2

Lakeshore Greenway

SCENERY: ★ ★ ★ ★
TRAIL CONDITION: ★ ★ ★ ★
CHILDREN: ★ ★ ★
DIFFICULTY: ★ ★
SOLITUDE: ★

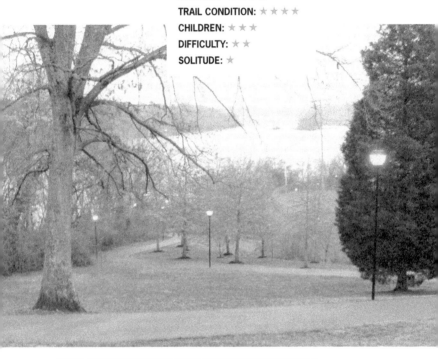

VIEWS OF THE TENNESSEE RIVER STRETCH TO THE HORIZON.

GPS TRAILHEAD COORDINATES: N35° 55.430' W83° 59.397'

DISTANCE & CONFIGURATION: 2.1-mile loop

HIKING TIME: 1.2 hours

HIGHLIGHTS: Incredible river and mountain views, loop greenway

ELEVATION: 920 feet at trailhead to 815 feet along river

ACCESS: No fees, passes, or permits required; open dawn to dusk

MAPS: Lakeshore Greenway, USGS Knoxville

FACILITIES: Restrooms and drinking fountains near ball fields

WHEELCHAIR ACCESS: Yes, for entire trail

COMMENTS: Loop has no greenway connections

CONTACTS: Knoxville Parks and Recreation, Lakeshore Park, 6414 South Northshore Dr., Knoxville, TN 37919; (865) 215-4311; **ci.knoxville.tn.us/parks**

Overview

The river and mountain views will impress first-time visitors to this 60-acre park, located astride a state-run mental-health institute. Start atop a hill overlooking the Tennessee River, then drop alongside Knoxville's master waterway, gaining aquatic vistas before turning up Fourth Creek and exploring the attractive rolling grounds of the historic facility.

Route Details

The notion of creating a park on the grounds of a downsized mental-health facility was hard to swallow for some, but it has turned out to be a great idea. Lakeshore is a state-run center that serves the mental health needs of East Tennesseans. It opened as East Tennessee Hospital for the Insane in 1886, then became known as Eastern State Mental Hospital. The place had a less-than-sterling reputation, as mentally ill Tennesseans were housed on the prison-like grounds with little rehabilitation taking place. Such were the times, and the bad rap stayed long after the place was downsized and modernized. The grounds themselves, located on a hill above and along Fourth Creek, are stunning and today would go for big bucks. Lakeshore Park was established in 1995, and this 2.1-mile greenway runs along the perimeter of the grounds. The asphalt trail is used by walkers and joggers who want to enjoy not only the views but also the hills that add extra zing to their exercise regimen. The trail also travels past many buildings of the institute, some of which are not being used. Expect to see Lakeshore Institute downsized more, with the park expanding.

Leave the parking area, heading east along a hill. First-rate panoramas of East Tennessee open in moments, including a long sweep of the Tennessee River, revealing the Smoky Mountains rising over the water. What a view! Park benches beckon here, and a few cedars border the track. At 0.1 mile, the Lakeshore Greenway switchbacks off the hill under planted oaks and cedars to saddle alongside the Tennessee River, which is dammed as Fort Loudon

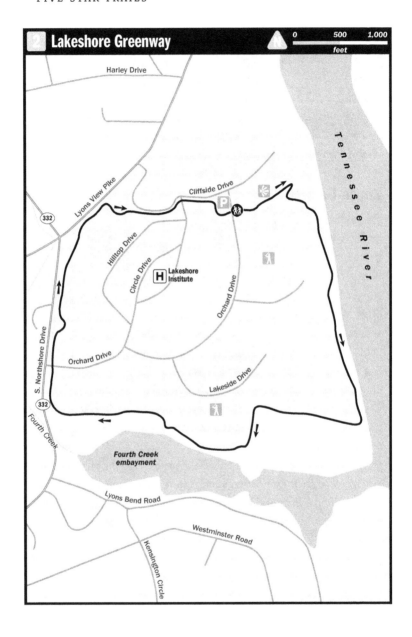

Lake at this point. On the downside, the trail is fenced from the water. The path is mostly open to the sky overhead as you pass beside ball fields. At 0.7 miles, the path turns west, away from the river and along the Fourth Creek embayment. Look for waterfowl in the shallows. The trail is marked in quarter-mile increments as it continues to skirt the property's outer edge. Pass planted sycamores lining the track. The entire greenway is lighted, allowing for sunrise and sunset walks, if you are so inclined.

At 1.1 miles, the trail makes a short but very steep incline, only to level out again. Cruise past institute buildings that have outlived their usefulness. Meet up with Northshore Drive at 1.3 miles. The Lakeshore Greenway continues its loop, now heading north. Bisect an alternate property entrance at 1.5 miles. Get ready for a good hill, which then levels off. Ahead, the white stone memorials of East Tennessee State Veterans Cemetery are visible across Lyons View. The cemetery for Lakeshore is nearby, where patients were interred after passing away. At one time Lakeshore was also used for patients with illnesses such as tuberculosis, as well as what is today known as Alzheimer's. Most of the 4,000 Lakeshore internee graves are unmarked.

Continue an uptick while turning away from Lyons View. At 1.9 miles, come alongside the park entrance road. The greenway seemingly stops, but cross a parking lot and then rejoin the path as it curves under a magnolia tree to complete the loop at 2.1 miles.

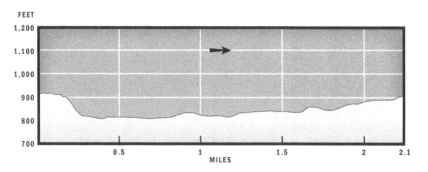

Directions

From Exit 383 (Papermill Drive) on I-40 in Knoxville, follow Papermill Drive 0.3 miles to reach Northshore Drive. Turn left on Northshore, southbound to cross Kingston Pike. Keep south beyond Kingston Pike 0.8 miles to reach Lyons View at a light. Turn left on Lyons View and follow it 0.3 miles to the right turn into Lakeshore Institute with a sign indicating Lakeshore Greenway. Enter the grounds, passing a stop sign at 0.2 miles. Keep forward beyond the sign, passing buildings on your right to reach the greenway parking area on your right.

3

Neyland Greenway

SCENERY: ★ ★ ★
TRAIL CONDITION: ★ ★ ★ ★ ★
CHILDREN: ★ ★ ★ ★ ★
DIFFICULTY: ★
SOLITUDE: ★

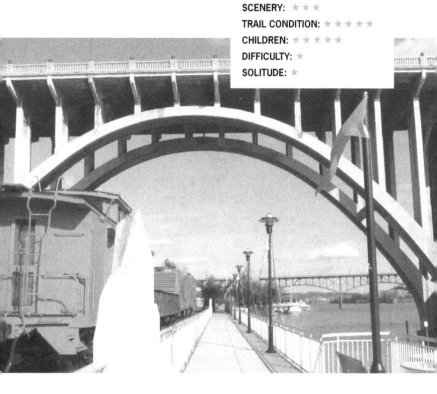

VOLUNTEER LANDING IS A POINT OF PRIDE FOR KNOXVILLIANS.

GPS TRAILHEAD COORDINATES: N35° 35.651' W84° 12.510'

DISTANCE & CONFIGURATION: 3-mile out-and-back

HIKING TIME: 1.5 hours

HIGHLIGHTS: City views, lake views

ELEVATION: 835 feet at trailhead to 850 feet at high point

ACCESS: No fees, permits, or passes required

MAPS: Neyland Greenway, USGS Knoxville

FACILITIES: Water, restrooms, riverside benches at trailhead

WHEELCHAIR ACCESS: Yes, for entire greenway

CONTACTS: Knoxville Parks and Greenways, 400 Main St., Knoxville, TN 37902; (865) 215-4311; **ci.knoxville.tn.us/parks**

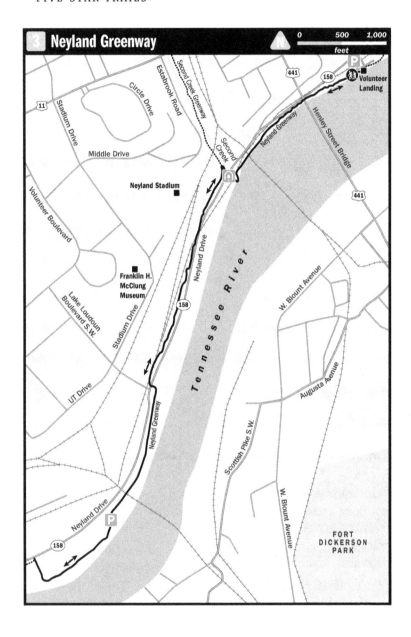

Overview

This downtown greenway starts at Volunteer Landing, off Neyland Drive astride the Tennessee River, where an alluring trailhead makes for a great pre- or post-hiking relaxation venue. Head west on the greenway along the river before tunneling under Neyland Drive at the Second Creek Greenway. Continue down Neyland Drive, passing iconic Neyland Stadium before returning to the river to soak in views of the Cherokee Bluffs across the water and then backtracking. Keep in mind this is an urban trek involving a road crossing and city sounds and sights. Also, this greenway connects to other trails, potentially adding mileage to this outing.

Route Details

Neyland Greenway is a scenic urban path and an important connector that links several other paved paths in Knoxville's ever-expanding city trail system. This trek starts at downtown's Volunteer Landing, one of many developed areas along the Neyland Greenway. Volunteer Landing is a brick structure overlooking the Tennessee River. It has restrooms, water, and benches, all designed for enjoying the riverside scenery. Restaurants and entertainment are all within easy walking distance of Volunteer Landing. Downtown Knoxville is up the hill from the river. Pick up the greenway and travel westerly,

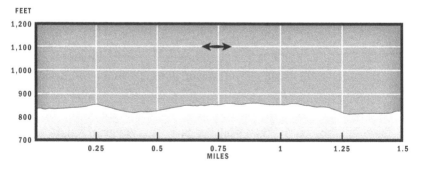

away from Calhoun's Restaurant. Enjoy views of the Tennessee River and the land rising across the water. Soon enter an area with many artsy fountains where kids play in summer. The concrete walkway is bordered with attractive iron railings and lampposts. Interpretive signage delivers historical vignettes detailing Knoxville's longtime relationship with the Tennessee River, the reason for the city's being here in the first place. The stuff is really fascinating. Take the time to read up on and visualize the many incarnations of the area where you walk.

Railroad tracks, Neyland Drive, and boats on the river remind you this area has long been a transportation corridor. The greenway is yet another venue as walkers, bikers, and Rollerbladers ply the concrete track. Volunteers fans even access it to attend University of Tennessee sporting events. Boat landings are used by visitors and the Vol Navy, an impromptu flotilla of University of Tennessee football devotees who voyage the river to see the Big Orange in action. Pass under the historic arched Henley Street Bridge and then under a utilitarian railroad bridge at 0.3 miles. Ahead, come to an intersection. Here, the Neyland Greenway curves left over the river at the UT Rowing Club Building, then tunnels under Neyland Drive along Second Creek. Once on the north side of Neyland Drive, you reach a greenway intersection. Here, the Second Creek Greenway heads north along Second Creek to World's Fair Park.

You take the now-asphalt Neyland Greenway up the north side of Neyland Drive and pass Neyland Stadium, home of the University of Tennessee football Volunteers. Keep along the drive, passing in the shadow of Thompson-Boling Arena (where the men and women Vols play basketball) to reach Lake Loudon Boulevard and a traffic light at 0.9 miles. Cross Neyland Drive using the traffic crosswalk, then resume the greenway, now back along the Tennessee River. Enjoy views of boaters and rowers on nice days. At 1.2 miles, travel under another railroad bridge. The path then turns away from Neyland Drive, passing an alternate parking area with just a few spaces, as well as the public Neyland Drive boat ramp.

The greenway then circles behind a City of Knoxville water treatment plant. A wooden boardwalk extends over rock riprap on the water. The Cherokee Bluffs rise 250 feet across the river. This is a favorite spot for river lovers. At 1.5 miles, the Neyland Greenway returns to Neyland Drive. This is a good place to turn around. However, you can continue along the greenway for 0.4 miles to reach the Third Creek Greenway, which makes other connections. Also, if you want to extend your trek in the other direction, the Neyland Greenway heads east from Volunteer Landing, where you started, to meet the James White Greenway, which heads north to Morningside Park.

Nearby Attractions

The Women's Basketball Hall of Fame is just down the road. Check out the history of women's basketball through the decades in this city where the Tennessee Lady Volunteers continue to set the standard of greatness. For more information visit **wbhof.com.**

Directions

From Exit 388A on I-40, take James White Parkway, southbound, then veer onto the Neyland Drive Exit from James White Parkway. Neyland Drive soon comes along the Tennessee River. Turn left into Volunteer Landing at a traffic light. Cross the railroad tracks and turn right for parking. The left turn for parking is for Calhoun's Restaurant.

Northwest/Victor Ashe Greenway

SCENERY: ★ ★ ★
TRAIL CONDITION: ★ ★ ★ ★
CHILDREN: ★ ★ ★
DIFFICULTY: ★
SOLITUDE: ★

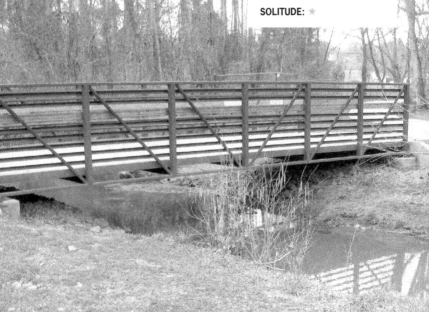

THIS GREENWAY WANDERS OVER HILL AND STREAM.

GPS TRAILHEAD COORDINATES: N35° 59.356′ W83° 59.973′

DISTANCE & CONFIGURATION: 3.4-mile double loop

HIKING TIME: 1.8 hours

HIGHLIGHTS: Pond and stream, two parks

ELEVATION: 980 feet at trailhead to 1,040 feet at high point

ACCESS: No fees, permits, or passes required; open dawn to dusk

MAPS: Northwest Greenway, USGS Bearden, Knoxville

FACILITIES: Restrooms at Victor Ashe Park

WHEELCHAIR ACCESS: Yes for entire trail

CONTACTS: Knoxville Parks and Recreation, Northwest Middle Park, 5301 Pleasant Ridge Rd., Knoxville, TN 37912; (865) 215-4311; ci.knoxville.tn.us/parks

Overview

This greenway trek connects Northwest Middle Park to Victor Ashe Park. Leave Northwest Park to travel along Third Creek, passing springs and crossing the stream to reach Victor Ashe Park, a large open green space. Enjoy a pair of ponds, then make a loop on the Victor Ashe Greenway before backtracking to Northwest Middle Park, where you complete a second loop.

Route Details

Victor Ashe was Knoxville's longest-serving mayor, holding office for 15 years from 1988 to 2003. A strong proponent of parks, Mr. Ashe not only doubled the city's park acreage from 700 to more than 1,700 but also saw to it that more than 30 miles of greenways were laid down. Thus it was fitting to name a park and a greenway after the honorable mayor. Now we can enjoy the fruits of Ashe's labor. This trek starts at Northwest Middle Park, a 15-acre green space shared with Northwest Middle School. The asphalt track first makes a loop before you leave Northwest Middle Park. You then pick up a connector trail along the upper stretches of Third Creek and enjoy a riparian zone centered by the rushing stream and also some springs that pop up in the wetlands adjacent to the stream. The connector takes you to Victor Ashe Park, a sizable 115-acre preserve with plenty of room to roam. You will then reach the loop and developed facilities of Victor Ashe Park before backtracking to your point of origin.

In the afternoon during the school year you may see students walking or running around the short loops at Northwest Middle Park. Nearby residents will be there too. Join a slender asphalt track heading back toward Pleasant Ridge Road. Come very near Pleasant Ridge Road before circling around a playground and gazebo. Turn away from Pleasant Ridge Road. The loop splits at 0.3 miles. Stay right, soon coming along wooded Third Creek. Pass picnic shelters and tennis courts to leave the park at 0.5 miles. Cross Walpine Lane and pick up the connector path linking Northwest Middle Park to Victor

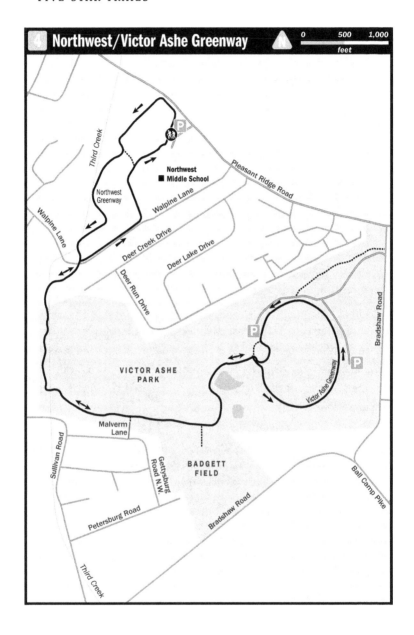

Northwest/Victor Ashe Greenway

N

0   500   1,000
feet

Third Creek

Northwest
■ Middle School

Pleasant Ridge Road

Northwest
Greenway

Walpine Lane

Walpine Lane

Deer Creek Drive

Deer Lake Drive

Deer Run Drive

Bradshaw Road

VICTOR ASHE
PARK

Victor Ashe Greenway

Malvern
Lane

Sullivan Road

Gettysburg
Road N.W.

BADGETT
FIELD

Ball Camp Pike

Petersburg Road

Bradshaw Road

Third Creek

Ashe Park, which widens to 10 feet. Travel under hardwoods as you bridge Third Creek at 0.7 miles. Note the clear springs flowing into the main stream. The trail is concrete in this area to better withstand periodic flooding, which is sure to occur. Bridge Third Creek again at 0.8 miles. Cane grows thick near the waterway.

Cross the driveway of a residence at 0.9 miles, then enter Victor Ashe Park, a mix of field and forest. The grassy hills were once grazed by cattle. Views of the surrounding wooded ridges are revealed as you undulate on the higher hills. At 1 mile, a short connector path leads right to Malvern Lane and a neighborhood. These connectors attract local residents to utilize their public parks. At 1.2 miles, another connector path leads right to Badgett Fields, a ball field complex. Note the huge cedar trees at this trail junction. These are likely relics from when this area was farmland. They were perhaps planted along a fence line at least a century ago. The trail curves past a pair of ponds. Visitors attracted to the green space of this large park invariably congregate here. The pond also lures anglers.

At 1.4 miles, reach the Victor Ashe Greenway. Stay right here and begin circling around ball fields to reach the developed area of Victor Ashe Park, with restrooms, picnic shelters, and the like. Victor Ashe Park is accessed off Pleasant Ridge Road from Bradshaw Road. At 1.9 miles, a spur trail leads right, to the park entrance. Shortly, you'll complete the loop of Victor Ashe Greenway and then begin

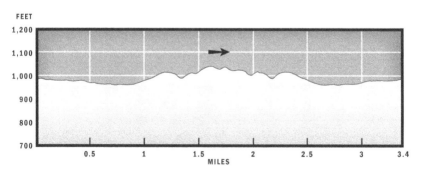

backtracking toward Northwest Middle Park. Enjoy more views beyond the fields before reaching Third Creek again at 2.7 miles. The wooded stream environment contrasts greatly with the open fields of Ashe Park.

Cross Walpine Lane a second time at 3 miles and enter Northwest Middle Park. This time stay right, completing the portion of this loop you didn't do before, staying closer to Northwest Middle School. Complete the loop at 3.4 miles.

Nearby Attractions

Victor Ashe Park has ball fields, open space, picnic shelters, a dog park, and a renowned disc golf course.

Directions

From Exit 108 (Merchants Drive) on I-75 north of Knoxville, take Merchants Drive west, passing under I-75, and follow it for 2.1 miles to intersect Pleasant Ridge Road. Turn left on Pleasant Ridge Road and travel just a short distance before turning right into Northwest Middle School, which is also the parking area for the park. The asphalt track starts on your right.

Third Creek Greenway

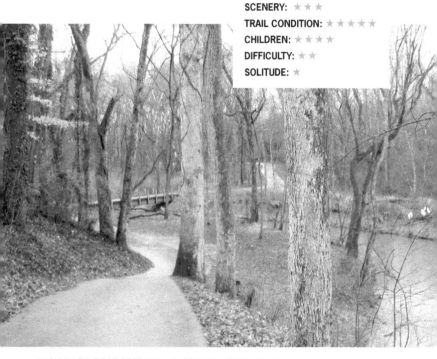

SCENERY:	★ ★ ★
TRAIL CONDITION:	★ ★ ★ ★
CHILDREN:	★ ★ ★
DIFFICULTY:	★ ★
SOLITUDE:	★

KNOXVILLE'S FIRST GREENWAY IS STILL AN ATTRACTION.

GPS TRAILHEAD COORDINATES: N35° 57.238' W83° 56.531'

DISTANCE & CONFIGURATION: 3.6-mile out-and-back

HIKING TIME: 2 hours

HIGHLIGHTS: Wooded creekside environment, developed park at trailhead

ELEVATION: 825 feet at trailhead; 885 feet at turnaround point

ACCESS: No fees, passes, or permits required; open dawn to dusk

MAPS: Knoxville Mega Greenway, USGS Knoxville

FACILITIES: Picnic area, restrooms, and other recreation facilities at Tyson Park

WHEELCHAIR ACCESS: Yes, for entire trail

COMMENTS: Greenways extend in both directions from this hike.

CONTACTS: Knoxville Parks and Recreation–Tyson Park, 2351 Kingston Pike, Knoxville, TN 37916; (865) 215-4311; **ci.knoxville.tn.us/parks**

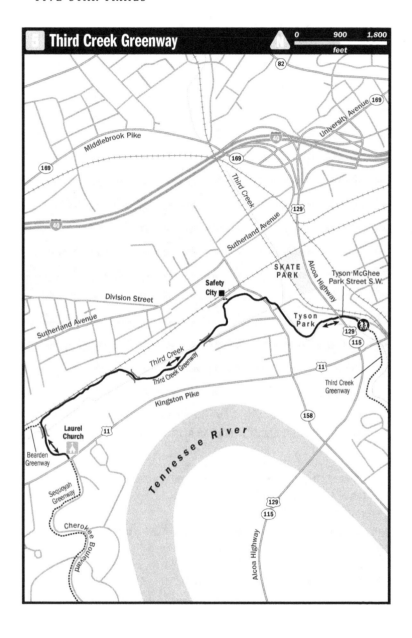

Overview

This hike near the University of Tennessee (UT) campus travels the main connector line for the Knoxville greenway system. Third Creek Greenway, Knoxville's oldest linear park trail, leaves Tyson Park and travels west along Third Creek. Swaddled in woods, making it a good summertime trek, the paved path occasionally crosses its namesake stream while traveling a few hills before turning south and making a final climb for Kingston Pike, where it connects with the Sequoyah Greenway.

Route Details

Third Creek Greenway began to take form in the 1970s, which makes it the oldest greenway in Knoxville. Of course, back then it was referred to simply as Third Creek Bike Trail, before the term "greenway" came into vogue. Knoxville developed the trail at the behest of the American Heart Association. The path started near Tyson Park and went westerly to Painter Avenue. I used it as a UT student in the 1980s. It has since expanded in both directions and has been connected with other Knoxville greenways to become the primary east-west connector for a trail system that can lead hikers, bicyclists, and joggers from near Northshore Road in Bearden east to

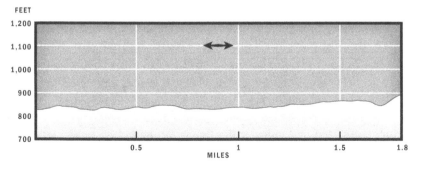

James White Parkway downtown. Look for more expansions on what has become Knoxville's Mega Greenway!

Pick up the Third Creek Greenway at the southeastern end of Tyson Park, near the Kingston Pike entrance. The trail continues south from Tyson Park to meet the Neyland Greenway 1 mile distant at the Tennessee River, but this hike heads northwest to pass under the bridge of busy Alcoa Highway, then enters the bulk of Tyson Park. Third Creek flows over rocks to your left, draining points north that flow to the Tennessee River. The stream gains its name from being the third creek west of where Knoxville was settled, in what is now downtown, with First Creek being the aquatic point of settlement. Second Creek has a greenway too. It travels through Worlds Fair Park.

Third Creek Greenway hugs Third Creek across from a bluff as it cruises past the developed facilities of Tyson Park. Knoxville's second-oldest green space, behind Chilhowee Park, was named for the first Tennessee plane pilot killed in battle, McGhee Tyson, who perished over the North Sea during World War I. Curve past a playground, turning north to leave Tyson Park at 0.4 miles. Bridge a tributary of Third Creek just as you reach Concord Street. The greenway then crosses Concord and enters Third Creek Park, a wooded corridor, sometimes wide, sometimes narrow, but a swath nonetheless, offering a natural respite amid civilization. At 0.6 miles, a spur trail leaves right and uphill for Safety City, a place where elementary students are schooled in pedestrian safety, fire safety, and more, complete with traffic signals; it's a quasi-training area. The main greenway veers left, bridging a wetland and Third Creek before coming to a spur path leading left to Painter Avenue at 0.8 miles.

The asphalt track descends a hill to a wooded picnic area. Note the trailside granite blocks denoting the community members who donated land for the project. The path undulates not only up and down but also left and right, adding pleasant meanderings. Third Creek chatters downstream in small shoals and rapids. Occasional gravel bars afford stream access. You will bridge Third Creek again at 1.1

miles. You are now on the right-hand bank of Third Creek. A wooded wetland spreads around the stream, and the trail is pushed against a railroad line, looking for higher ground. The first rail line using Third Creek Valley was the Knoxville Belt Railway, built in the 1880s. The aspiring loop around the city was only partially constructed. The line you see today is the Norfolk Southern.

At 1.5 miles, the greenway reaches a junction. Here, the main path keeps straight 1.4 miles to Bearden, with a shorter spur heading to Sutherland Avenue. This hike travels left to span Third Creek one more time before making a solid climb under tall trees to end at the parking lot of Laurel Church on Kingston Pike at 1.7 miles. A water fountain is nearby. Across the street, the Sequoyah Greenway begins its 2.6-mile one-way journey through a well-heeled neighborhood and along the Tennessee River. Large riverside Sequoyah Park attracts area residents. But to keep this round-trip walk to 3.6 miles, your best bet is to backtrack to the trailhead, though you can walk east along Kingston Pike to make a loop. However, the sounds and scenery won't match that of Third Creek.

Nearby Attractions

Tyson Park has picnic shelters, tennis courts, a playground, and ball fields.

Directions

From Exit 386B on I-40 near UT, take US 129 south to shortly exit at Kingston Pike, US 11/US 70. Turn left, eastbound toward UT. Travel 0.1 mile to turn left into Tyson Park. Follow the park road just a short distance to a parking area on your left under shade trees. Pick up the greenway here.

Will Skelton Greenway

SCENERY: ★ ★ ★ ★
TRAIL CONDITION: ★ ★ ★ ★ ★
CHILDREN: ★ ★ ★ ★

GPS TRAILHEAD COORDINATES:
N35° 57.335' W83° 52.099'

DIFFICULTY: ★ ★
SOLITUDE: ★ ★

DISTANCE & CONFIGURATION:
4.2-mile out-and-back

HIKING TIME: 2.2 hours

HIGHLIGHTS: River views, wildlife management area

ELEVATION: 865 feet at trailhead; 845 feet at turnaround point

ACCESS: No fees, permits, or passes required; open dawn to dusk

MAPS: Will Skelton Greenway, USGS Shooks Gap

FACILITIES: Restrooms and water fountain at Ijams Nature Center

WHEELCHAIR ACCESS: Yes, for entire trail

COMMENTS: Trailhead is at Ijams Nature Center, which has hiker-only trails.

CONTACTS: Knoxville Parks and Recreation–Ijams Nature Center, 2915 Island Home Ave., Knoxville, TN 37920; (865) 215-4311: **ci.knoxville.tn.us/parks**

Overview

This paved trek leaves Ijams Nature Center using the Will Skelton Greenway to enter Forks of the River Wildlife Management Area, a natural setting of woodland and meadow. Cruise along the inception of the Tennessee River, then curve up the French Broad River to end at a bluff offering elevated views of the French Broad and beyond. Some hills add to the challenge, while creeks add more watery scenery.

Route Details

Will Skelton is a well-known conservationist icon of Knoxville parks, greenways, and the general outdoors scene. Active both locally and nationally in the Sierra Club, he was an instrumental part of the Cherokee National Forest Wilderness Coalition, which helped set aside roadless areas in Tennessee's only national forest. He even edited a book about the trails of the Cherokee. A lawyer by trade,

Skelton championed building greenways in Knoxville, serving as the chairman of the Knoxville Greenways Commission, so it is only fitting that such a scenic path would be named for him.

The Will Skelton Greenway, popular with walkers, bicyclists, and joggers, begins at Island Home Park, then travels easterly to reach Ijams Nature Center, where this hike picks up the path. Enjoy traveling through nature center property, then bisect a brief section of "civilization" to enter the wildlife management area that presents a natural scene for you to enjoy.

From the nature center entrance, head southeast on a 10-foot-wide asphalt track. Island Home Avenue is to your right. The trail immediately passes a solar energy capture station that helps fuel the Ijams Nature Center visitor building. Immediately enter lush woods, then make a downward curve. Traverse an old railroad track near Mead's Quarry, which is visible to your right, southwesterly, then at 0.4 miles bridge Toll Creek, which gurgles its way to meet the Tennessee River. At this point, you will leave Ijams Nature Center property.

The trail then turns sharply east as it parallels McClure Lane. Here, the path exhibits characteristics more typical of an urban greenway, a track paralleling houses and businesses. However, this section is short-lived as, at 0.8 miles, the greenway leaves McClure Lane and bridges a creek to come alongside the Tennessee River.

Enter the Forks of the River Wildlife Management Area (WMA), managed by the Tennessee Wildlife Resources Agency. The name Forks of the River refers to the three rivers that come together at this point. The French Broad River has cut easterly through the mountains from North Carolina, while the Holston River has come from the coal country of southwestern Virginia. Both rivers travel a fair distance through the Volunteer State, and it is here their waters meet to form the Tennessee River. The WMA offers a green landscape of open fields and cedar and hardwood forests, along with wetlands and the riparian zone that borders the Tennessee and French Broad rivers. It is amazing that this 605-acre tract of wilderness lies so close to downtown Knoxville. You may see wildlife that calls this area home.

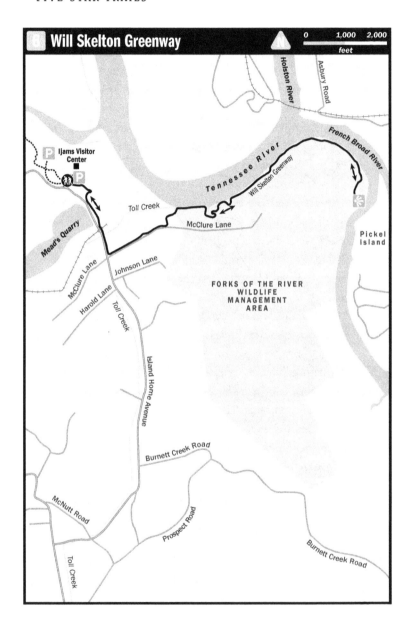

Hikers will commonly spot deer and wild turkeys, while birders can enjoy not only songbirds but also shorebirds along the river and raptors overhead. Birders have counted more than 175 species at Forks of the River WMA. Be apprised that this wildlife management area is intermittently open to hunting between September and February. However, the greenway remains open for use.

At 1 mile, bridge another stream, arguably the uppermost tributary on the entire Tennessee. Here, the trail doubles back on itself before coming back alongside the water. Hardwoods partially shade the trail. At 1.3 miles, come alongside a large open field to your right, while a screen of vegetation lies between you and the Tennessee. Some fields are being used to grow crops for wildlife, while others have been periodically burned to restore native grasses.

At 1.6 miles, reach the spot where you can look upon the three rivers at once. See if you notice different water coloration between the French Broad and the Holston. The trail stays along the river's edge, but it has now joined the French Broad, where barges and industry are visible across the river. The easy, level cruise ends at 2 miles. The greenway turns away from the water and climbs to reach a bluff—the trail terminus—at 2.1 miles. Here, you can gaze up the valley of the French Broad. Pickel Island splits the river in the foreground. A resting bench beckons. From here, backtrack 2.1 miles to the trailhead to complete your hike at 4.2 miles.

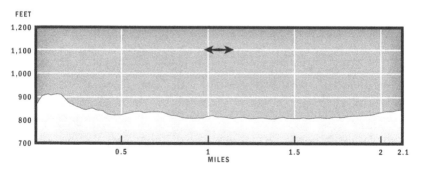

Nearby Attractions

Other hiking opportunities branch out from the trailhead. From the Ijams entrance, the Will Skelton Greenway extends westerly 1.2 miles to Island Home Park, and Ijams Nature Center has plenty of trails, including the hike described in this book on page 20.

Directions

From the intersection of Cumberland Avenue and Gay Street in downtown Knoxville, travel south over the Tennessee River on the Gay Street Bridge to reach the traffic light. Keep forward at the light, now on Sevier Avenue. Travel 0.6 miles on Sevier Avenue, then stay left on Island Home Avenue as Sevier Avenue curves right over railroad tracks. Stay on Island Home Avenue for 2 miles to reach Ijams Nature Center on your left. Park immediately upon entering the nature center. Pick up the Will Skelton Greenway near the Ijams entrance gate.

William Hastie Natural Area

SCENERY: ★ ★
TRAIL CONDITION: ★ ★ ★
CHILDREN: ★ ★ ★
DIFFICULTY: ★ ★
SOLITUDE: ★ ★ ★

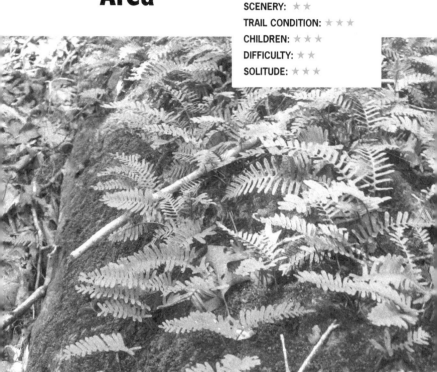

WATCH FOR INTIMATE NATURAL BEAUTY AT WILLIAM HASTIE NATURAL AREA.

GPS TRAILHEAD COORDINATES: N35° 56.079' W83° 52.470'

DISTANCE & CONFIGURATION: 2.6-mile loop

HIKING TIME: 1.4 hours

HIGHLIGHTS: Deep woods, rock ledges and outcrops

ELEVATION: 960 feet at trailhead to 1,060 feet at high point

ACCESS: No fees, permits, or passes required; open dawn to dusk

MAPS: William Hastie Natural Area, USGS Shooks Gap, Knoxville

FACILITIES: Picnic table and shelter

WHEELCHAIR ACCESS: None

CONTACTS: Knoxville Parks and Recreation, 400 Main St., Knoxville, TN 37902; (865) 215-4311; **ci.knoxville.tn.us/parks**

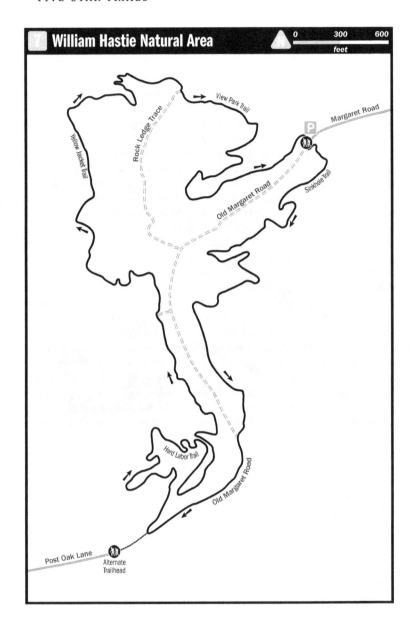

William Hastie Natural Area

0   300   600
feet

View Park Trail

Margaret Road

Rock Ledge Trace

Yellow Jacket Trail

P

Old Margaret Road

Sinkhole Trail

Hard Labor Trail

Old Margaret Road

Post Oak Lane

Alternate
Trailhead

Overview

This loop hike travels through a 75-acre tract of hilly wilderness located in suburban South Knoxville. Once a farm, the rugged terrain, full of rock outcrops and sinkholes amid dense woodland, offers nearly 4 miles of trails developed by a local mountain biking club. Hikers are more than welcome on the trails, which can be a quick escape for those desiring a deep-woods connection with nature.

Route Details

What a great addition to the Knoxville park system! William Hastie Natural Area contrasts greatly with typical urban parks, with their playgrounds, ball fields, and paved trails. This destination is an old hardscrabble farm reverted to wooded wildland, where natural-surface trails explore darn near every nook and cranny of the tract. You will be surprised at the steep and rugged topography—and wonder how anybody could've ever farmed it. But farm they did.

John Chandler grew up near the trailhead. In 1947, his family bought 97 acres, along with the house, which had no running water, no electricity, and outdoor bathrooms. They collected roof runoff and drained it into a cistern for storage. The family lived off some livestock and a garden, eventually adding lights and water. Chandler was 1 of 13 children raised here during the 17 years they called what is now

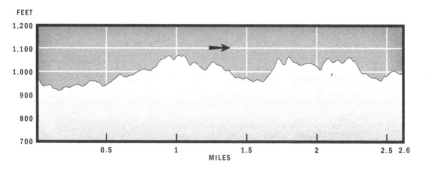

William Hastie Natural Area home. As you hike, imagine 13 kids, plus cows, pigs, and chickens running around these now-thick woods.

Three trails split from the Margaret Road trailhead. While facing the big boulders blocking Old Margaret Road, head left past the picnic shelter on Sinkhole Trail. Old Margaret Road continues past the boulders, while View Park Trail leaves to the right. The slender singletrack Sinkhole Trail shortly enters woods, where many walnut trees stand overhead. Cruise the edge of a hollow with a rocky cedar-covered hill rising to your left.

When hiking, keep an eye and ear open for mountain bikers. They built the trails and bridges we hike. Pass over a trio of bridges at 0.2 miles. The path is generally easy to follow except where it crosses old farm roads and where people shortcut switchbacks. Just stay with the most-used singletrack and you will be fine. (Copy the map from this book just in case.)

Meet Old Margaret Road at 0.7 miles. Turn left on the gravel track, traveling the base of a hollow whereupon tulip tree–covered hills rise to a point where you wouldn't begin to guess that the park is surrounded by houses. The many sinkholes here prevent continual running water in the streambeds. At 0.8 miles, the Hard Labor Trail leads acutely right. Ahead, Old Margaret Road leads a short distance to meet the Post Oak neighborhood entrance to the natural area.

Stay with the Hard Labor Trail as it winds up a hillside to reach what was likely an old rock quarry. Climb into dogwoods and pines, reaching a high point at 1.1 miles. Begin a convoluted, twisted course using tight switchbacks that prevent erosion and maximize mileage in the limited space of the natural area. Note the elongated rock outcroppings and rock piles beside the path. In winter these outcrops will stand out. In spring the hollows will show off their share of wildflowers.

Descend to meet the Yellow Jacket Trail at 1.6 miles. A short path leads right to Old Margaret Road. Keep straight, joining the singletrack Yellow Jacket Trail, heading northerly and bridging a couple of streambeds to make another trail junction at 2.2 miles.

Here, the Rock Ledge Trail leaves to the right. This loop stays left, crossing an old roadbed to pick up the singletrack View Park Trail. This path makes long, loping switchbacks down a south-facing rock, hickory, and cedar hill. Descend gently, drifting into the trailhead at 2.6 miles, to complete the loop hike.

Nearby Attractions

The natural area offers more trails in addition to the loop described. Old Margaret Road Trail cuts through the heart of the natural area and connects to all the other paths. It follows the low point of the main valley. Rock Ledge Trail winds along a hillside limestone outcrop. These trails add more loop possibilities should you want to go a different route on a second or third trip here.

Directions

From Exit #388A on I-40 east of downtown Knoxville, take James White Parkway south 3.2 miles to the Moody Avenue exit. Exit James White Parkway, then turn left, crossing over the parkway, to join Sevierville Pike. Follow Sevierville Pike 1.8 miles on a very winding road to a right turn onto Margaret Road. Follow Margaret Road 0.3 miles to dead-end in a parking area.

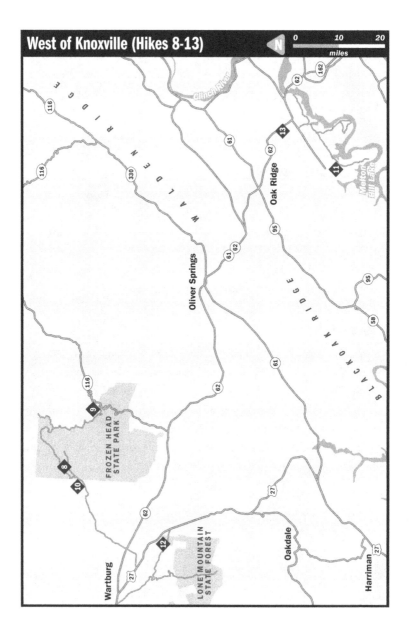

West of Knoxville (Hikes 8-13)

West

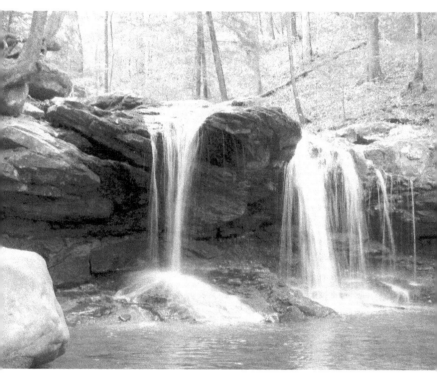

FROZEN HEAD STATE PARK IS ONE OF KNOXVILLE'S NEARBY NATURAL ASSETS.

Frozen Head State Park:
Emory Gap Falls and DeBord Falls

SCENERY: ★ ★ ★ ★
TRAIL CONDITION: ★ ★ ★
CHILDREN: ★ ★ ★
DIFFICULTY: ★ ★
SOLITUDE: ★ ★ ★

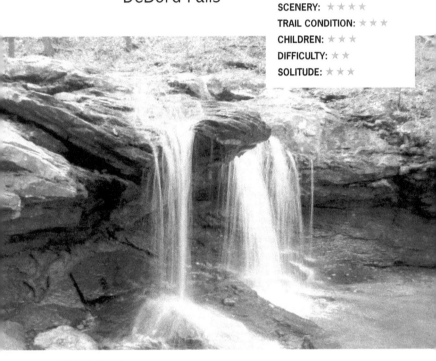

DEBORD FALLS

GPS TRAILHEAD COORDINATES: N36° 8.200' W84° 29.254'

DISTANCE & CONFIGURATION: 2.8-mile out-and-back

HIKING TIME: 1.8 hours

HIGHLIGHTS: Three waterfalls, Cumberland Mountains

ELEVATION: 1,520 feet at trailhead to 1,990 feet at turnaround point

ACCESS: No fees, permits, or passes required; open year-round, daily, 8 a.m.–sunset

MAPS: Frozen Head State Park, USGS Fork Mountain

FACILITIES: Restrooms, water fountains, camping, visitor center

WHEELCHAIR ACCESS: None

CONTACTS: Frozen Head State Park, 964 Flat Fork Rd., Wartburg, TN 37887;
(423) 346-3318; **tnstateparks.com**

Overview

This waterfall hike in mountainous Frozen Head State Park leads to two named cascades as it explores a rugged valley carved from the highest terrain on the entire Cumberland Plateau. The hike is easier than you might think because it follows an old roadbed most of its distance. Traveling along North Prong Flat Fork, the hike enters a wildflower-laden valley to reach DeBord Falls, complemented by a shaded pool. The ascent sharpens upon joining Emory Gap Branch, where Emory Gap Falls drops over a stone lip framed by a rock house.

Route Details

The road leading to the trailhead passes an attractive picnic area. Consider bringing a pre- or post-hike meal on your Frozen Head State Park adventure. The Panther Branch parking area has a turnaround at the uppermost part, but do not park in the turnaround. Panther Branch Trail passes a trailside kiosk, then immediately bridges North Prong Flat Fork. Sycamore, hemlock, and buckeye shade the stream as it flows over smooth rocks. Beech, black birch, and tulip trees rise up the valley.

Before you know it a spur trail veers right to an unnamed waterfall spilling into Flat Fork. This modest tributary cascade tumbles off the north side of Old Mac Mountain, dropping over layers of rock before adding its flow to Flat Fork. Like many of the watercourses here at Frozen Head, this stream may run nearly dry in late summer and fall. The wide path traverses intermittent streambeds flowing off Bird Mountain to your left, north. Bird Mountain and Old Mac Mountain together create the valley through which North Prong Flat Fork flows.

Unlike most other trails at Frozen Head, this path makes for easy hiking because it follows an old jeep road. Therefore, you can focus on your surroundings rather than watching every footfall. Also, hikers can walk side by side, conversing as they travel. Occasional large boulders stand in the stream and among the woods around you.

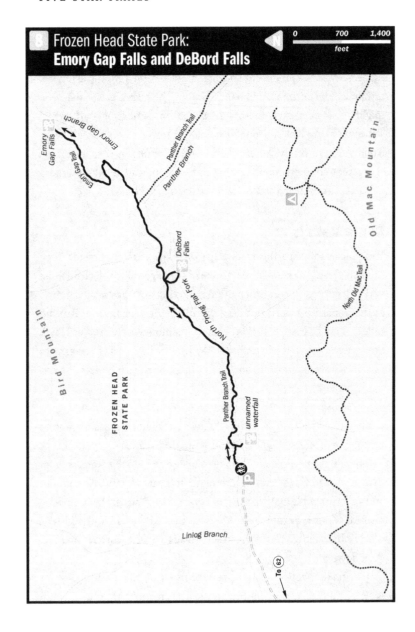

Frozen Head State Park:
Emory Gap Falls and DeBord Falls

0   700   1,400
feet

Emory Gap Branch

Emory Gap Falls

Emory Gap Trail

Panther Branch Trail

Panther Branch

Old Mac Mountain

DeBord Falls

North Prong Flat Fork

North Old Mac Trail

Bird Mountain

FROZEN HEAD STATE PARK

Panther Branch Trail

unnamed waterfall

P

Linlog Branch

To 62

Small trees sometimes find a home atop more level boulders. Keep an eye out for exposed bluffs overlooking the creek. Pass a deep, alluring pool at 0.3 miles. This is a great place for kids to play in the water and ruin their new hiking boots. The ascent picks up at 0.5 miles. Bridge a branch at 0.6 miles, then come to the spur loop leading to DeBord Falls. Here, take a short trail leading to a bluff-top overlook of the cascade. Ahead, steps lead to the base of the falls, which drops 15 feet over a jagged rock ledge into a gravel-bordered pool. A sturdy hemlock stands in repose by DeBord.

Continue up Panther Branch Trail, shortly bridging another intermittent streambed. At 0.9 miles, Panther Branch Trail leaves to the right up Panther Branch to meet North Old Mac Trail. This hike, however, keeps straight, joining Emory Gap Trail, ascending along Emory Gap Branch. The hike still traces an old jeep road that makes a pair of switchbacks at 1.1 miles, heading deeper into the mountain valley. Bridge another intermittent streambed at 1.2 miles. Saddle alongside Emory Gap Branch as it flows through large gray boulders, obscuring the flow and giving the impression of a watercourse that is more rock than water.

Travel along the edge of a tall rock house. Emory Gap Falls is visible in the distance. Pick your way carefully upstream through a boulder garden bordered by the rock house on one side and Emory Gap Branch on the other. Reach the falls at 1.4 miles. Several user-created

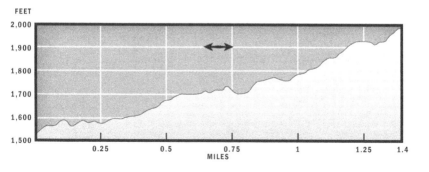

trails approach the falls from different directions, as hikers attempt to gain the best vantage. The tall cataract spills over a rock ledge, framed on one side by the rock house and the other side by a wooded hill. Don't climb atop the falls—the mossy rocks are slick and invite disaster. Photographers will be challenged to compose the varied landscape here, with the boulder garden, the rock house, surrounding woods, and waterfall. The pool below the falls is somewhat shallow, as Emory Gap Branch is a generally low-flowing creek. Your legs will enjoy the 500-foot descent back to the trailhead to complete the 2.8-mile trek much more than they liked the climb.

Nearby Attractions

Frozen Head State Park offers not only hiking but also fishing, camping, and nature study on its 21,000 acres of wildlands. Also, a segment of the Cumberland Trail travels through the park.

Directions

From Knoxville, take Pellissippi Parkway toward Oak Ridge, joining TN 62 west to reach Oliver Springs. From Oliver Springs, follow TN 62 west 13 miles to turn right onto Flat Fork Road. A sign for Morgan County Regional Correctional Facility and Frozen Head State Park alert you to the right turn. Follow Flat Fork Road 4 miles to the entrance of Frozen Head State Park. The visitor center is on your right. Keep straight, passing the main hiker trailhead. Continue left for 1 mile beyond the main trailhead, passing the campground spur road to dead-end at the Panther Branch trailhead.

Frozen Head State Park:
Frozen Head Tower via Armes Gap

SCENERY: ★ ★ ★ ★
TRAIL CONDITION: ★ ★ ★ ★
CHILDREN: ★ ★
DIFFICULTY: ★ ★ ★
SOLITUDE: ★ ★ ★ ★

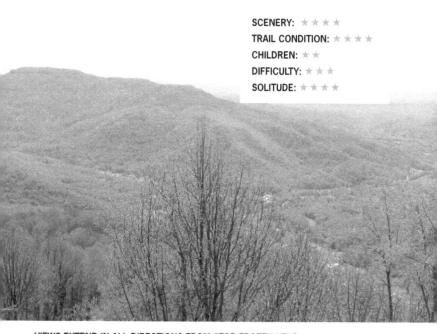

VIEWS EXTEND IN ALL DIRECTIONS FROM ATOP FROZEN HEAD.

GPS TRAILHEAD COORDINATES: N36° 6.985' W84° 26.355'

DISTANCE & CONFIGURATION: 5.4-mile out-and-back with option of additional 0.8-mile out-and-back to prison mine

HIKING TIME: 4 hours

HIGHLIGHTS: 360-degree view from observation tower, historic prison mine

ELEVATION: 2,100 feet at trailhead to 3,324 feet at high point

ACCESS: No fees, permits, or passes required; open year-round, daily, 8 a.m.–sunset

MAPS: Frozen Head State Park, USGS Petros

FACILITIES: None

WHEELCHAIR ACCESS: None

COMMENTS: Frozen Head State Park has more than 30 miles of hiking trails in addition to this hike.

CONTACTS: Frozen Head State Park, 964 Flat Fork Road, Wartburg, TN 37887; (423) 346-3318; **tnstateparks.com**

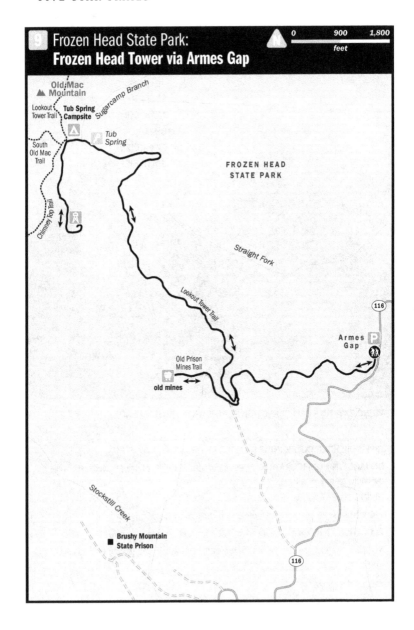

9 Frozen Head State Park: Frozen Head Tower via Armes Gap

0   900   1,800
feet

Old Mac Mountain

Lookout Tower Trail
Tub Spring Campsite

Sugarcamp Branch

Tub Spring

South Old Mac Trail

Chimney Top Trail

FROZEN HEAD STATE PARK

Straight Fork

Lookout Tower Trail

116

Armes Gap

Old Prison Mines Trail

old mines

Stockstill Creek

Brushy Mountain State Prison

116

Overview

This trail takes you to the highest point on the Cumberland Plateau, Frozen Head Mountain, standing at 3,324 feet. Here, an observation tower allows a 360-degree view from the boundaries above Frozen Head State Park. On a clear day you can look east across the Tennessee River Valley to the Smoky Mountains and west across the plateau as far as the clarity of the sky allows. This route is the shortest with the least amount of elevation gain, but it still climbs a solid 1,200 feet. Add a historic component by visiting the old Brushy Mountain Prison Mine on your way back.

Route Details

Lookout Tower Trail passes around a metal gate and heads southwest from Armes Gap. The gated doubletrack is open only to official vehicles. TN 116 will be on your left and is visible through the trees. You are expecting a climb, but it starts out pretty easy, picking up steam at 0.3 miles. A rich hardwood forest dominated by hickory, tulip, maple, and oak shades the gavel-and-dirt path. At 0.7 miles, reach a split. Here, Old Prison Mines Trail leads left on a level doubletrack, while Lookout Tower Trail continues ascending. Save the Old Prison Mines Trail for your return trip after scaling Frozen Head.

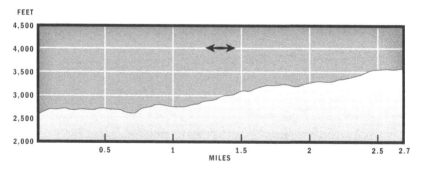

65

On the way in you pass Brushy Mountain State Prison, a fortress-like facility established in 1896. Its most famous inmate was James Earl Ray, convicted of assassinating Martin Luther King Jr. in Memphis. Ray escaped from Brushy Mountain in the 1970s but was quickly recaptured. The penitentiary is reserved for the state's most hardened criminals, but don't let this deter you from undertaking the hike, as escapes are exceedingly rare. I have camped overnight 30 or more times in the backcountry of Frozen Head State Park and slept peacefully every hour of darkness.

Beyond the intersection, Lookout Tower Trail makes a hard switchback to the right. At 0.9 miles, the path crosses over to the right-hand (north) side of the mountain. Views open on Big Fodderstack Mountain to the east. This ridgeline marks the Tennessee Valley Divide. Streams to the north and east flow into the Cumberland River, while streams to the south and west feed the Tennessee River. Pass a small grassy clearing and keep ascending, as Frozen Head rises sharply to your left. Springs flow over rock outcrops in the forest above you.

More wintertime views open to the northeast. The trail continues curving up the mountain, turning sharply west at 1.9 miles. The climbing eases as you pass Tub Spring, enclosed in stone to your left at 2.2 miles. Drift into a major trail junction. Tub Spring Campsite lies up a small hill to your right. Lookout Tower Trail splits here. One leg heads right and downhill to the state park campground, while the other leg turns left to the crest of Frozen Head. Other trails spur from here to lace Frozen Head State Park. Stay left toward the tower, still climbing on a doubletrack. Curve around the south side of the peak. The observation tower and radio towers come into view. Reach the top of Frozen Head at 2.7 miles. Here, an old apple tree grows next to radio towers. Steps lead to an open observation platform built on the infrastructure of a historic fire tower. From the observation platform you can look west into the valley of Flat Fork and beyond. To the northeast the mountains of Catoosa Wildlife Management Area ripple to the horizon. To the southeast lies Petros, Brushy Mountain Prison, and the Tennessee River Valley. On a clear day the Smoky Mountains are visible and a practiced eye can easily identify the peaks of Mount LeConte.

From the tower, backtrack 2 miles to the Old Prison Mines Trail. Here, turn right and follow a grassy doubletrack westerly, for a total of 0.4 miles. This old roadbed is much less used than the trail to the tower. Shortly you'll pass by a very small clearing and continue on a level path to enter another more open field after 0.3 miles. Next pass beneath an old stone wall and come to the first mine opening. You can look into the stone maw—through bars—and see the wooden beams that help stabilize the mine. Prisoners once hand-dug coal beneath Frozen Head, and the mines operated until the 1960s. An old railroad tram led down the mountain to the prison. Imagine the toiling that went on here. Continue past this first mine entrance to a couple more openings, bordered by concrete with an old concrete block guard shack nearby. These were obviously the newer mines. This is your turnaround point. Explore but don't enter the shafts—only a fool enters abandoned mines. Backtrack to the Lookout Tower Trail, returning to Armes Gap after a total hike of 6.2 miles, including the 0.8-mile round-trip segue on the Old Prison Mines Trail.

Nearby Attractions

Frozen Head State Park offers not only hiking but also fishing, camping, and nature study on its 21,000 acres of wildlands. Also, a segment of the Cumberland Trail travels through the park.

Directions

From Knoxville, take Pellissippi Parkway toward Oak Ridge, joining TN 62 west to reach Oliver Springs. From Oliver Springs, follow TN 62 west 8.1 miles to TN 116. Look for signs to Petros. Turn right on TN 116 north and travel 4.6 miles, passing through Petros and by Brushy Mountain Prison to Armes Gap. The hike starts on the west side of the gap, to your left, as you drive from Petros.

Frozen Head State Park:
Judge Branch Loop

SCENERY: ★ ★ ★ ★
TRAIL CONDITION: ★ ★ ★ ★
CHILDREN: ★ ★ ★ ★ ★
DIFFICULTY: ★ ★
SOLITUDE: ★ ★ ★ ★

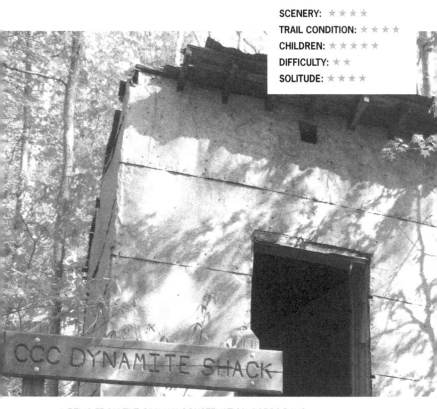

A RELIC FROM THE CIVILIAN CONSERVATION CORPS DAYS

GPS TRAILHEAD COORDINATES: N36° 7.626' W84° 30.021'

DISTANCE & CONFIGURATION: 2.9-mile loop

HIKING TIME: 1.8 hours

HIGHLIGHTS: Mountain stream, wildflowers, bluff

ELEVATION: 1,390 feet at trailhead to 1,790 feet at turnaround point

ACCESS: No fees, permits, or passes required; open year-round, daily, 8 a.m.–sunset

MAPS: Frozen Head State Park, USGS Fork Mountain, Petros

FACILITIES: Restrooms, water fountains, camping, visitor center

WHEELCHAIR ACCESS: None

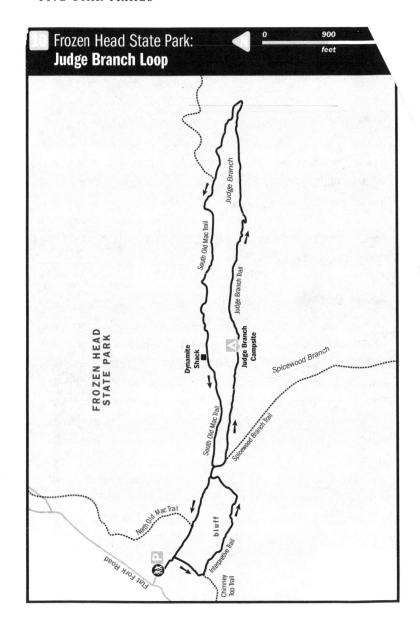

Frozen Head State Park:
Judge Branch Loop

0   900
feet

Judge Branch

South Old Mac Trail

Judge Branch Trail

**FROZEN HEAD
STATE PARK**

**Dynamite
Shack**

**Judge Branch
Campsite**

Spicewood Branch

South Old Mac Trail

Spicewood Branch Trail

North Old Mac Trail

bluff

Interpretive Trail

Flat Fork Road

Chimney Top Trail

COMMENTS: Frozen Head State Park has more than 30 miles of hiking trails in add
this hike.

CONTACTS: Frozen Head State Park, 964 Flat Fork Rd., Wartburg, TN 37887;
(423) 346-3318; **tnstateparks.com**

Overview

This valley loop hike is one of the best wildflower destinations in the
greater Knoxville area as it travels up the Judge Branch watershed into
the heart of Frozen Head State Park. Start the trek on an interpretive
trail before reaching Judge Branch Trail. Lush woods border the clear
stream with everywhere-you-look beauty. Wildflowers burst forth in
April, and spring is the most popular time to hike this relatively easy
loop that is great for all ages.

Route Details

Bring your wildflower identification book on this hike. You will do
well, especially if you hit the trail in April. The peak wildflower time
varies year to year, so call the park office in early spring to fine-tune
your wildflower trek. Park rangers actually lead wildflower hikes at
Frozen Head if you want to go that route. Judge Branch Loop is
still a good hike year-round for families and people of all ages who
want a taste of the mountains without biting off more than they
can chew.

Morgan County, site of the state park, was settled in the
early 1800s by simple German farmers. Later, rich coal and timber
resources were extracted. The logging era ended in the 1920s, and
Frozen Head was bought by the state and declared Morgan Forest
Reserve. The reserve was transferred to the state parks department
in 1970. The park's recreational stature has grown, and it is now a
lauded hiking and camping destination, with 19 campsites bordering
Big Cove Branch and Flat Fork. The level sites are set amid large
boulders that give them a distinctive Cumberland Mountains feel.
Consider complementing your Frozen Head State Park experienc

COMMENTS: Frozen Head State Park has more than 30 miles of hiking trails in addition to this hike.

CONTACTS: Frozen Head State Park, 964 Flat Fork Rd., Wartburg, TN 37887; (423) 346-3318; **tnstateparks.com**

Overview

This valley loop hike is one of the best wildflower destinations in the greater Knoxville area as it travels up the Judge Branch watershed into the heart of Frozen Head State Park. Start the trek on an interpretive trail before reaching Judge Branch Trail. Lush woods border the clear stream with everywhere-you-look beauty. Wildflowers burst forth in April, and spring is the most popular time to hike this relatively easy loop that is great for all ages.

Route Details

Bring your wildflower identification book on this hike. You will do well, especially if you hit the trail in April. The peak wildflower time varies year to year, so call the park office in early spring to fine-tune your wildflower trek. Park rangers actually lead wildflower hikes at Frozen Head if you want to go that route. Judge Branch Loop is still a good hike year-round for families and people of all ages who want a taste of the mountains without biting off more than they can chew.

Morgan County, site of the state park, was settled in the early 1800s by simple German farmers. Later, rich coal and timber resources were extracted. The logging era ended in the 1920s, and Frozen Head was bought by the state and declared Morgan Forest Reserve. The reserve was transferred to the state parks department in 1970. The park's recreational stature has grown, and it is now a lauded hiking and camping destination, with 19 campsites bordering Big Cove Branch and Flat Fork. The level sites are set amid large boulders that give them a distinctive Cumberland Mountains feel. Consider complementing your Frozen Head State Park experience

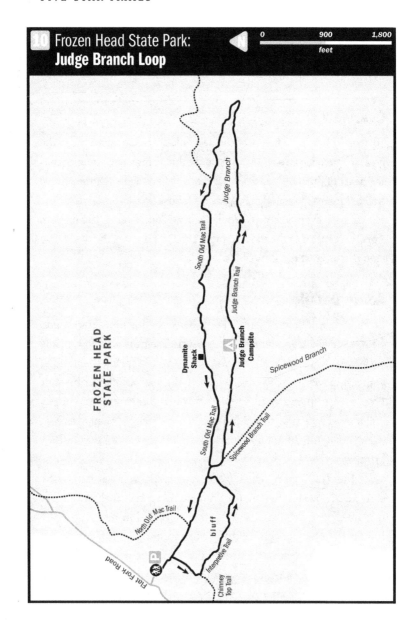

with camping. Hot showers and water spigots add a touch of civilization to the natural amenities.

The trailhead parking area offers a picnic shelter, restrooms, and water. Leave the trailhead, joining an easterly path that travels just a few feet to reach a trail junction. Here, the Interpretive Trail and Chimney Top Trail leave to the right. Turn right here on the Interpretive Trail, traveling south through level woods to shortly reach Judge Branch. Chimney Top Trail keeps straight, bridging Judge Branch, while the Interpretive Trail curves left, upstream along Judge Branch. Soon look left for the old holding tanks of a fish hatchery built by the Civilian Conservation Corps, who developed the park in the 1930s. You may have noticed the trailside monument honoring three of the young corps members who perished during that time. Continue up the hemlock-dominated valley, looking for a sheer rock bluff on the far side of the stream. The Interpretive Trail curves away from Judge Branch to reach a trail junction at 0.5 miles. Turn right here and shortly meet South Old Mac Trail, which leaves left for Tub Spring and the high country. Keep straight before angling south toward Judge Branch, which you soon cross on a bridge.

Just ahead, the Spicewood Branch Trail branches right, also bound for the high country. Stay left on Judge Branch Trail, traveling deeper into the wildflower-carpeted valley. Judge Branch gurgles over a rocky bed, sometimes gathering in pools and other times spilling

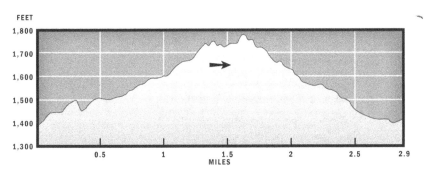

in shoals. Tall white oaks, sweetgums, smooth beeches, stately red maples, and black birch shade the path. Watch for the hand-cut stone drainage culverts astride the trail—more handiwork from the CCC boys. Dwarf crested iris, phlox, halberd-leaved violets, trilliums, Solomon's seal, and other wildflowers will color the forest floor in April. At 0.7 miles, cross Spicewood Branch on a footbridge. Note the rockwork on the bridge here as well.

Continue east up the valley, reaching the spur trail to Judge Branch campsite at 1 mile. The spur leads left to a hemlock-shaded flat overlooking Judge Branch. Non-campers could use it as a picnic spot. Back on the main trail look for ferns aplenty as well as sycamores close to the stream. Bridge a tributary at 1.1 miles. The ascent is gentle but steady. Reach stone steps that take you down to Judge Branch at 1.4 miles. Here, the valley has steepened and you must rock-hop the creek, an easy proposition under normal flows. The eye-pleasing locale beckons a stop. Ample boulders and stones make good sitting spots.

Turn back downstream among big boulders in more rugged terrain. Rock sentinels rise above the path. Walk just below a low-flow slide cascade, then pass another dripping falls to meet South Old Mac Trail on a south-facing oak and mountain laurel slope at 1.7 miles. Keep west on the slender singletrack path. Judge Branch is audible below. At 2.2 miles, pass the old Civilian Conservation Corps dynamite shack. Explosives were stored here during the park development. The dynamite was used to fashion park roads and trails. Ahead, walk around a conspicuous boulder in the path; it surely came to rest here since the CCC days. South Old Mac Trail ends at 2.5 miles. Turn right here, following the well-used, 0.4-mile path that shortly passes the Interpretive Trail and North Old Mac Trail before returning to the parking area.

Nearby Attractions

Frozen Head State Park offers not only hiking but also fishing, camping, and nature study on its 21,000 acres of wildlands. Also, a segment of the Cumberland Trail travels through the park.

Directions

From Knoxville, take Pellissippi Parkway toward Oak Ridge, joining TN 62 west to reach Oliver Springs. From Oliver Springs, follow TN 62 west 13 miles to turn right onto Flat Fork Road. A sign for Morgan County Regional Correctional Facility and Frozen Head State Park alert you to the right turn. Follow Flat Fork Road 4 miles to the entrance of Frozen Head State Park. The park visitor center is on your right. Keep straight beyond the visitor center, shortly turning into the main hiker trailhead on your right.

Gallaher Bend Greenway

SCENERY: ★ ★ ★ ★

TRAIL CONDITION: ★ ★ ★

CHILDREN: ★ ★

DIFFICULTY: ★ ★ ★

SOLITUDE: ★ ★ ★

GPS TRAILHEAD COORDINATES: N35° 57.390' W84° 14.982'

DISTANCE & CONFIGURATION: 4-mile balloon loop

HIKING TIME: 2.1 hours

HIGHLIGHTS: Lushly wooded trailside, Melton Hill Lake vistas

ELEVATION: 810 feet at trailhead to 920 feet at high point

ACCESS: No fees, permits, or passes required; open dawn to dusk

MAPS: Gallaher Bend Greenway, USGS Bethel Valley, Lovell

FACILITIES: Restrooms, drinking fountains, swim area, boat ramp at Clark Center Park

WHEELCHAIR ACCESS: Yes, for entire trail

COMMENTS: No pets allowed

CONTACTS: Oak Ridge Recreation and Parks Department,1403 Oak Ridge Turnpike, Oak Ridge, TN; (865) 425-3453; **orrecparks.org**

Overview

Don't let the moniker "greenway" mislead you. This trek travels through a wooded wildlife management area on a gravel track deep into a bend on the Clinch River, here dammed as Melton Hill Lake. Gallaher Bend, located on the Oak Ridge Reservation, is part of the Three Bends, a wildlife preserve of more than 3,000 acres. The trail itself wanders hills and past fields and woods to reach a vista of Melton Hill Lake.

Route Details

This hike will smash your notions of a greenway. It should be called a trail. The trek leaves Clark Center Recreation Park, which offers picnicking, boating, and swimming, then enters a wildlife management area managed by the Tennessee Wildlife Resources Agency (TWRA). Gallaher Bend is a wildlife-rich area, where deer, turkey, waterfowl, and game birds enjoy habitat that includes upland woods, fields sown for wildlife, and fields containing native grasses, hedgerows, and miles of shoreline on Melton Hill Lake. The reason this area is still wild is due to its being on the Oak Ridge Reservation, federally held land acquired by the U.S. government during the days when Oak Ridge was a secret city, working on the atomic bomb. The reservation has been in their hands for seven-plus decades, and civilization has sprung up around it, leaving a de facto nature preserve. Today, the area is governed under the auspices of the Department of Energy (DOE), but TWRA does the actual land management for the area. It is also used for environmental research by the University of Tennessee and the DOE.

On any given day you will find walkers, hikers, and bicyclists traveling from Clark Center Park deep into Gallaher Bend. During the cooler months, the last 0.3 miles of the road leading to the trailhead may be gated, so prepare to add that distance to your hike. Be sure to check the TWRA hunt schedule before you go: **ornl.gov/sci/rmal/ huntinfo.htm.**

The trail starts just beyond the Clark Center Park swimming area on Melton Hill Lake. The gravel doubletrack trail enters a small hollow centered by a creek. Beech, pine-oak, and hickory woods shade the path. Gently climb the first 0.3 miles and open onto a mown field at 0.8 miles. Here, Gallaher Bend is at its narrowest, and you can see Melton Hill Lake to the northeast and southwest. The path is bordered by densely growing shortleaf pines, which indicates there was once more field than is visible today. The wide trail allows hikers to walk side by side, and the gravel bed lets you keep your eyes on the scenery rather than watch every footstep.

At 1.1 miles, the trail ascends again. Stone outcrops abut the path as a ridge rises to your left. Reach a gap at 1.4 miles and the high point of your hike, elevationally speaking. The trail levels off. Reach the loop portion of the trek at 1.6 miles. Here, an old road angles up to the left. This is part of the old Bull Bluff Road that you have been following. The hike, however, stays right on the gravel track and shortly opens to a field. Here, you can enjoy eye-popping panoramas

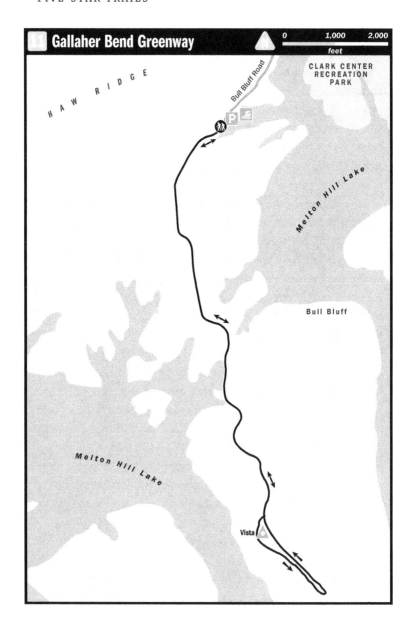

down riverine Melton Hill Lake. The Gallaher Bend Greenway makes one last dip before rising to end on a hill at 2 miles. You are nearly at the tip of Gallaher Bend. Oak Ridge Reservation gate 23J leads to a field, but this hike joins the primitive track that turns back toward the trailhead. Note the large trees lining the trail. Complete the loop portion of the hike at 2.4 miles. Backtrack 1.6 miles to the trailhead.

Directions

From Knoxville, take Pellissippi Parkway south toward Oak Ridge, joining TN 62 west. After crossing Melton Hill Lake on a bridge, watch for the Bethel Valley Road exit and join Bethel Valley Road, heading west to reach a traffic light. At the light, turn left on Pumphouse Road (the right turn here is Scarboro Road). Follow Pumphouse Road 0.3 miles, then turn right onto Bull Bluff Road, passing through a gate. At 1.8 miles, reach Clark Center Recreation Park. Continue forward a half mile to reach an outdoor swim area on your left. Park here. In winter the road will be gated 0.3 miles closer to the entrance of Clark Center Recreation Park.

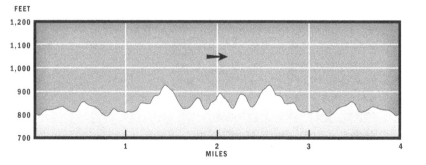

Lone Mountain State Forest Hike

SCENERY: ★ ★ ★
TRAIL CONDITION: ★ ★ ★
CHILDREN: ★ ★
DIFFICULTY: ★ ★ ★
SOLITUDE: ★ ★ ★

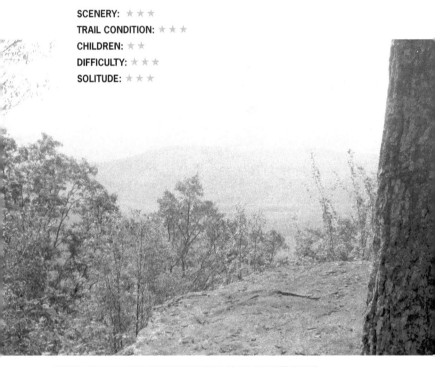

YOU'LL BE HOWLING ABOUT THE VIEWS FROM COYOTE POINT.

GPS TRAILHEAD COORDINATES: N36° 4.207' W84° 32.775'
DISTANCE & CONFIGURATION: 7.6-mile out-and-back
HIKING TIME: 4 hours
HIGHLIGHTS: Overlook at Coyote Point, Rankin Spring
ELEVATION: 1,370 feet at trailhead to 2,200 feet at high point
ACCESS: No fees, permits, or passes required; open dawn to dusk
MAPS: Lone Mountain State Forest, USGS Camp Austin
FACILITIES: Picnic table at trailhead, Rankin Spring, and Coyote Point
WHEELCHAIR ACCESS: None
CONTACTS: Lone Mountain State Forest, 302 Clayton Howard Rd., Wartburg, TN 37887; (423) 346-6655; **state.tn.us/agriculture/forestry**

Overview

Take a trek in a lesser-visited state forest, climbing the slopes of Lone Mountain to reach a rock outcrop and panoramic vista from Coyote Point. The climb is moderate, making it doable by anyone with patience and a decent set of lungs.

Route Details

Lone Mountain State Forest had long been on my hiking radar. And after going there for the first time, I wondered what took me so long to get there. Overshadowed by the nearby and popular Frozen Head State Park, Lone Mountain seems to have been forgotten by many hikers, though it does see some use by equestrians and mountain bikers.

Before 1970, Lone Mountain and Frozen Head both were part of the Morgan State Forest. Frozen Head was transferred to the state park system, while Lone Mountain remained part of the state forest. Some tracts of land were acquired by the state in the 1920s from landowner tax default. Another portion was purchased from the Lone Mountain Land Company, which had abused the property. The forest was allowed to regenerate for several decades and is now a scenic destination used by outdoor enthusiasts of all stripes, including hunters. If you are concerned about hiking while the area is being used for hunting, call the forest ahead of time to find out the exact dates.

An archway leads hikers from the trailhead into the state forest. A natural-surface path slices south through oak-holly-hickory woods. Bridge a tributary of Crooked Fork at 0.2 miles. Shortly, switchback up a ridgeline and then level off. You are expecting the trail to climb, but it doesn't quite yet. You may have to work around occasional muddy areas in the flats. At 1 mile, the trail joins the bulk of the mountain and curves westerly. Winter views open to the west through the leafless trees. Begin working your way up the east slope of Lone Mountain, entering a steep ravine, only to make a sharp switchback to the right at 1.5 miles. The climb eases and partial views open to the east toward Frozen Head.

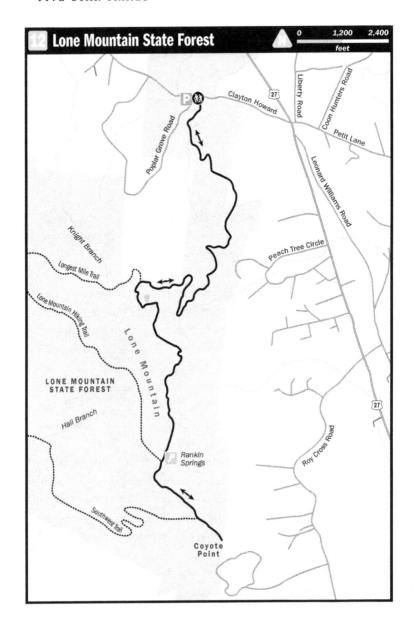

Swing around to the north side of Lone Mountain, cruising at an elevation of 1,900 feet. Intersect the Longest Mile Trail at 2.1 miles. It continues working westerly along the north slope of Lone Mountain under tulip trees, while the trail to Coyote Point turns left and continues uphill, making a pair of short switchbacks, back in drier forest of black gum and hickory. Pass a small pond to your left at 2.2 miles. By 2.4 miles, you have done nearly all your climbing and are cruising the easterly slope of Lone Mountain at an elevation of 2,100 feet. The peak of Lone Mountain rises to your right.

At 3.2 miles, reach Rankin Springs, a stone-lined watering hole that is also covered by an open-sided shelter. The water has never looked good here and is not recommended for drinking. However, the area has picnic tables, and there is also a small pond here. It makes a good stopping spot. Just ahead the simply named Hiking Trail—open to hikers only—leaves right and heads over the crest of Lone Mountain. Other area trails are open to hikers, mountain bikers, and equestrians. The Hiking Trail can be overgrown and is recommended for winter and spring hiking only. Lone Mountain State Forest has approximately 15 miles of trails open to visitors.

At 3.6 miles, the Southwest Trail leaves to the right for the lower slopes. Keep straight here, aiming for Coyote Point. At 3.8 miles, the terrain levels out and you open onto the grass, tree, and rock area of Coyote Point. The rock outcrop extends at the farthest

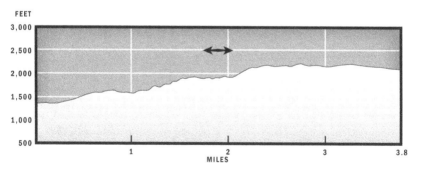

reach of the ridge, allowing you to step out and take in panoramas to the south and west. The cooling towers of Kingston Springs power plant are clearly visible. The bulk of the Cumberland Plateau rises to the west. On a clear winter day you can see the Smokies to the southeast. At this point you're probably wondering what took so long to get here also. Just be glad you're here, open your pack, and have a relaxing lunch or snack at the picnic tables situated at the overlook.

Nearby Attractions

Frozen Head State Park, just a few miles distant, makes a great camping base from which to explore the 15 miles of trails at Lone Mountain when you have time.

Directions

From Knoxville, take Pellissippi Parkway toward Oak Ridge, joining TN 62 west to reach Oliver Springs. From Oliver Springs, follow TN 62 west 10.5 miles to Petit Lane. Turn left and follow Petit Lane 1.7 miles to intersect US 27. Cross US 27 and continue straight, now on Clayton Howard Road. Follow Clayton Howard Road 0.4 miles and reach the trailhead on your left.

Oak Ridge Arboretum Loop

SCENERY: ★ ★ ★ ★
TRAIL CONDITION: ★ ★ ★ ★ ★
CHILDREN: ★ ★ ★ ★
DIFFICULTY: ★ ★
SOLITUDE: ★ ★ ★

GPS TRAILHEAD COORDINATES:
N35° 59.620' W84° 13.202'

DISTANCE & CONFIGURATION:
2.3-mile loop

HIKING TIME: 1.2 hours

HIGHLIGHTS: Outdoor education opportunities

ELEVATION: 875 feet at trailhead to 1,100 feet at high point

ACCESS: No fees, permits, or passes required; trails open 8:30 a.m.–sunset

MAPS: Arboretum Self-Guided Walking Trails, USGS Lovell

FACILITIES: Visitor center with restrooms

WHEELCHAIR ACCESS: None

COMMENTS: No pets and no picnicking

CONTACTS: UT Oak Ridge Forest and Arboretum, 901 South Illinois Ave., Oak Ridge, TN 37830; (865) 483-3571; **http://forestry.tennessee.edu/ORForest**

Overview

Enjoy a trail network near Oak Ridge at the University of Tennessee Arboretum. Hike interpretive nature trails, learning not only about the trees but also the ecosystem around you while exploring a variety of environments. Leave the visitor center and explore a hillside before descending to a creek and adjacent wetland. Rise to a high ridge, then work your way down to the trailhead. Allow plenty of time to enjoy the interpretive information.

Route Details

The Oak Ridge Arboretum is a 250-acre preserve within the greater 2,260-acre Oak Ridge Forest and is headquarters of the University of Tennessee Forest Resources Research and Education Center. Its mission is to establish, collect, and cultivate woody plants, as well as to provide open space for the public to study the forest, and finally to

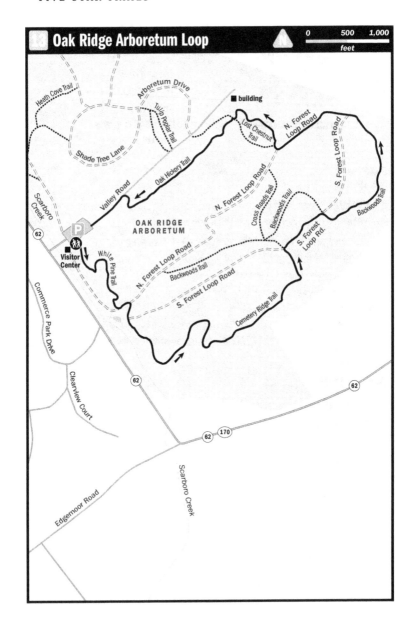

Oak Ridge Arboretum Loop

building

N. Forest Loop Road

Arboretum Drive

Heath Cove Trail

Tulip Poplar Trail

Lost Chestnut Trail

S. Forest Loop Road

Shade Tree Lane

Oak Hickory Trail

Valley Road

Scarboro Creek

N. Forest Loop Road

Cross Roads Trail

Backwoods Trail

S. Forest Loop Road

Backwoods Trail

62

OAK RIDGE ARBORETUM

Visitor Center

White Pine Trail

N. Forest Loop Road

S. Forest Loop Rd.

Backwoods Trail

S. Forest Loop Road

Cemetery Ridge Trail

Commerce Park Drive

Clearview Court

62

62

62

62 170

Edgemoor Road

Scarboro Creek

0   500   1,000
feet

provide a place to conduct plant-research programs. For the hiker this means a network of interpretive trails lacing the arboretum. Enjoy not only a fine walk in the woods but also an opportunity to absorb interpretive information about our native East Tennessee forests as well as exotic species. The arboretum also has a visitor center that complements the outdoor classroom.

Pick up the White Pine Trail near the visitor center, where trail maps are available, heading southbound. Busy TN 62 hums nearby. Cross a short footbridge and pass through a managed crabapple orchard while scaling a hillside. Enter full-blown woods. Note the lack of white pines here: they were wiped out during a pine beetle infestation. Dip to reach Marsh Road and Scarboro Creek at 0.3 miles. Look for the bald cypresses by Scarboro Creek. You will also find the central China collection, a group of trees transplanted from that country where the climate is similar to East Tennessee.

Turn left on North Forest Loop Road, then shortly curve right up South Forest Loop Road and join the Cemetery Ridge Trail within a short distance. The trail system is well marked and maintained with signs at every junction. Even though some of the trails are labeled as roads, they are used by park personnel only. All pathways are for hikers only. Contemplation benches are scattered throughout the trail system. The gravel Cemetery Ridge Trail climbs away from Scarboro Creek, then turns easterly, passing a sink to meet South Forest Loop

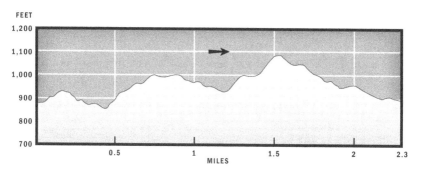

Road at 1 mile. Cross Roads Trail is dead ahead. This hike, however, turns right and travels easterly along South Forest Loop Road. At 1.2 miles, turn right on Backwoods Trail, roaming some of the most remote terrain in the arboretum. Dip to cross an intermittent streambed, then trek through a hickory-oak forest that was a field a century ago. The recuperative powers of nature are on display here.

A final climb leads to yet another trail junction near a TVA power line at 1.5 miles. Pick up the North Forest Loop Road, then angle away from the power lines, but not before enjoying a view of the Cumberlands created by the power line cut.

North Forest Loop Road leads you to another trail intersection at 1.7 miles. Turn right here, joining the Lost Chestnut Trail. Stay right as the Lost Chestnut Trail makes a loop of its own. This name comes from the trail's passing relic stumps from the mighty chestnut tree, which succumbed to blight. Personnel at this forest are involved in developing a strain of blight-resistant chestnuts. At 1.9 miles, look over a display about the chestnut. Keep straight, now on the Oak Hickory Trail, a singletrack path. Note the building below. The Oak Ridge Arboretum was established in 1964 and currently contains more than 2,500 native and exotic woody plant specimens. Interestingly, UT conducts on-site experiments in plant genetics (such as the one for the chestnut), insects and disease control, and general management of natural resources. This particular hike travels not only by many plant types but also through the associated different habitats. At 2.2 miles, the Oak Hickory Trail reaches Valley Road after descending stone and gravel steps. Turn left here, continuing downhill to reach the visitor center and complete your hike.

Directions

From Knoxville, take Pellissippi Parkway, TN 162, toward Oak Ridge, joining TN 62 west (South Illinois Avenue). After crossing Melton Hill Lake on a bridge, watch for the Bethel Valley Road exit. Pass the exit for Bethel Valley Road, then look for the signed entrance to the arboretum on your right.

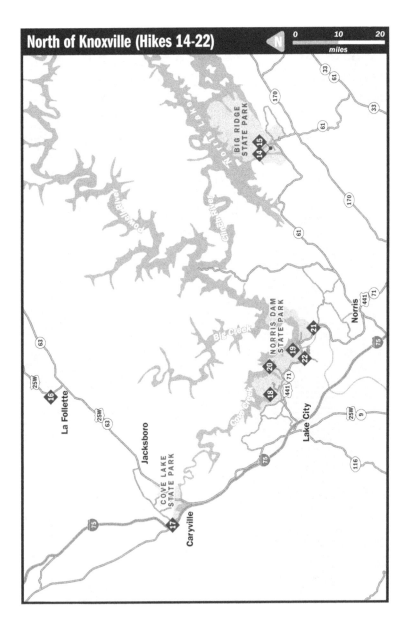

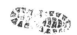 # North

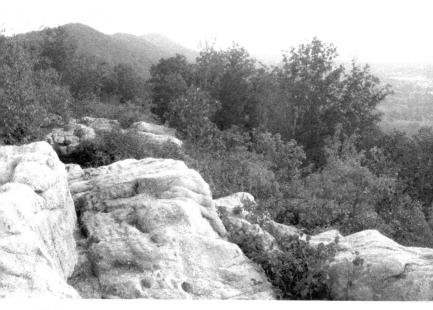

ATOP CUMBERLAND MOUNTAIN

14 # Big Ridge State Park:
Dark Hollow Loop

SCENERY: ★ ★ ★
TRAIL CONDITION: ★ ★
CHILDREN: ★ ★ ★
DIFFICULTY: ★ ★
SOLITUDE: ★ ★ ★

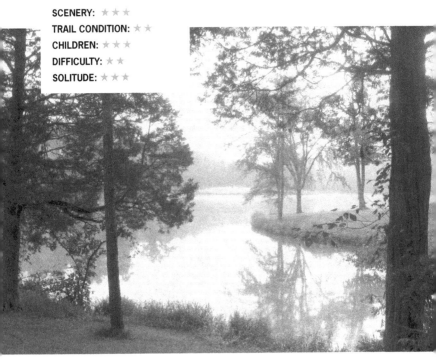

BIG RIDGE STATE PARK PRESENTS AQUATIC SPLENDOR.

GPS TRAILHEAD COORDINATES: N36° 14.595' W83° 55.883'

DISTANCE & CONFIGURATION: 5.5-mile balloon loop

HIKING TIME: 2.8 hours

HIGHLIGHTS: Two lakes, pioneer cemeteries, haunted trail

ELEVATION: 1,030 feet at trailhead to 1,380 feet at high point

ACCESS: No fees, permits, or passes required; year-round, daily, 8 a.m.–sunset

MAPS: Big Ridge State Park, USGS Big Ridge Park, White Hollow

FACILITIES: Restrooms and water fountain at nearby visitor center

WHEELCHAIR ACCESS: None

CONTACTS: Big Ridge State Park, 1015 Big Ridge Rd., Maynardville, TN 37807; (865) 992-5523; **tnstateparks.com**

Overview

This hike explores the human and natural history of Big Ridge State Park. Head out from the park lake and cross its dam. After traveling the shores of big Norris Lake, leave the water and enter Dark Hollow, where prepark pioneers toiled. Loop around to pick up Ghost House Trail, where you may have a haunting from one Maston Hutchinson, who is buried in a trailside cemetery. If you make it beyond the cemetery, rejoin the Lake Trail for more watery views. A short backtrack returns you to the trailhead.

Route Details

Big Ridge was one of Tennessee's first state parks. It was developed by the Civilian Conservation Corps (CCC) in conjunction with the building of Tennessee Valley Authority's first dam, creating Norris Reservoir. The park features rustic CCC stone construction. The lakeside setting of rugged ridge and valley country was once home to simple subsistence farmers. You can still see their homesites. Trails follow wagon roads they used. You can also see their cemeteries, one of which is the resting place of Maston Hutchinson, who is said to haunt the old road/trail that passes near his grave.

Enter the woods, heading north on the singletrack rock-and-dirt Lake Trail. Climb to reach the spur trail to Meditation Point at 0.1 mile. The Lake Trail meanders in mixed woods of pine, hickory, and oak hovering over the slender path, atop a steep ridge dropping off toward the park lake. At 0.4 miles, pass a covered bench. At 0.5 miles, the Loyston Overlook Trail leads left. It climbs a knob that offers winter views of Norris Lake. The Lake Trail saddles alongside the park lake, then reaches the dam that separates the park lake from Norris Lake. The park lake is generally kept at the same level, while Norris Lake is raised and lowered under the guidance of TVA. They factor in flood prevention, energy production, and recreation in their setting of Norris Lake levels.

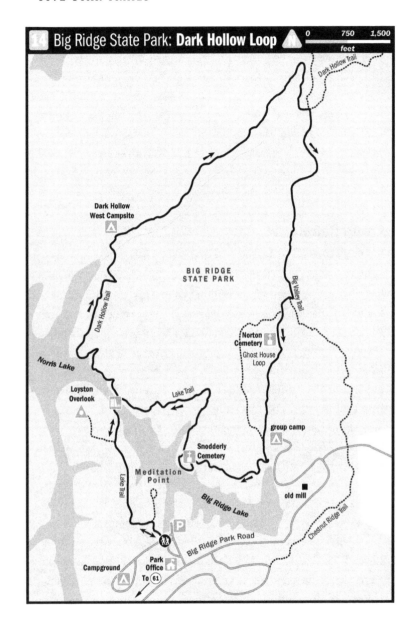

Reach the loop portion of the hike at 0.6 miles, heading left on the Dark Hollow Trail into mountain laurel, pines, and cedar. Skirt the shoreline of Norris Lake on a steep slope. What you see is the Bryant Fork arm of the impoundment, and it seriously belies the lake's true size. Circle a small embayment at 0.8 miles, then turn into Dark Hollow West embayment. Bridge the perennial unnamed stream flowing out of Dark Hollow West at 1.4 miles. Sycamores rise from the streambed. Turn into Dark Hollow to reach the Dark Hollow West backcountry campsite. It is located in a small hollow of Dark Hollow. Join an old wagon track bordered with sweetgum, dogwood, and pine. Look for faint roadbeds, stacked rocks, and other settler evidence as you penetrate deeper into the hollow. The path curves above the stream to reach a gap and four-way trail junction at 2.5 miles.

Turn right here, southbound on Big Valley Trail. Follow the old roadbed once used by subsistence farmers to haul corn to the Norton gristmill, located on a spring-fed stream that now feeds the park lake. Pass over Pinnacle Ridge, reaching a high point at 3 miles. Look for *beaucoup* beech trees up on this ridge, sure evidence that fire suppression has been in place for eight decades. Under natural, untamed circumstances, this number of beech trees would be found only in the moist hollows.

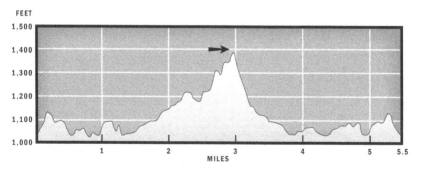

FEET

Descend from the high point to reach a trail junction at 3.2 miles. Head right, joining Ghost House Loop. Hopefully darkness isn't approaching. Just ahead, the trail splits; stay left, still on Ghost House Loop to reach the Norton Cemetery at 3.4 miles. Find the grave of Maston Hutchinson, who is the spirit responsible for the strange occurrences here and down trail at his old homesite, now known as the Ghost House. See if you can spot where the home once stood. Be very careful not to stray too far from the marked path.

Meet the other end of Ghost House Loop at 3.7 miles. Keep straight to meet the Lake Trail at 3.8 miles. A spur heads left to the group camp, but this hike turns right, circling the northeast side of the park lake, bridging two streamlets flowing off Pinnacle Ridge. Pass Snodderly Cemetery at 4.2 miles, uphill to your right. The path circles around a tributary, bridging it at 4.5 miles before returning to the park lake. Enjoy some final watery views before finishing the loop portion of the hike at 4.9 miles. Backtrack across the dam to complete the entire 5.5-mile hike. If you have any spare energy, climb to Loyston Overlook, then visit Meditation Point.

Nearby Attractions

The state park offers fishing, boating, and camping, in addition to hiking.

Directions

From Knoxville, take TN 33 north to TN 61. Follow TN 61 west 6.3 miles as it winds through hills to reach the state park on your right. Enter the park and drive a short distance to turn left at the old entrance station. The park office is to your left and offers maps. Continue downhill to park near the park lake. The trail starts on the road to the campground.

Big Ridge State Park:
Sharps Station Loop

SCENERY: ★ ★ ★
TRAIL CONDITION: ★ ★
CHILDREN: ★
DIFFICULTY: ★ ★ ★ ★
SOLITUDE: ★ ★ ★ ★

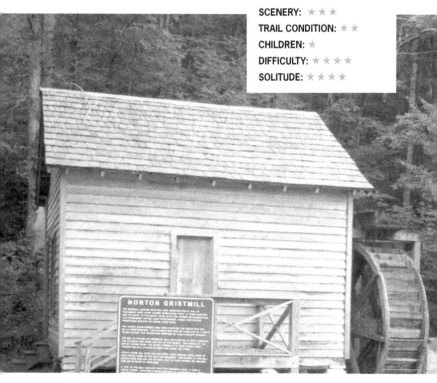

VISIT THIS MILL AT THE TRAILHEAD.

GPS TRAILHEAD COORDINATES: N36° 14.852' W83° 55.229'

DISTANCE & CONFIGURATION: 6.5-mile balloon loop

HIKING TIME: 4 hours

HIGHLIGHTS: Norris Lake, pioneer cemetery, historic site

ELEVATION: 1,060 feet at trailhead to 1,450 feet at high point

ACCESS: No fees, permits, or passes required; year-round, daily, 8 a.m.–sunset

MAPS: Big Ridge State Park, USGS Big Ridge Park, White Hollow

FACILITIES: Restrooms and water fountain at park visitor center

WHEELCHAIR ACCESS: None

CONTACTS: Big Ridge State Park, 1015 Big Ridge Rd., Maynardville, TN 37807; (865) 992-5523; **tnstateparks.com**

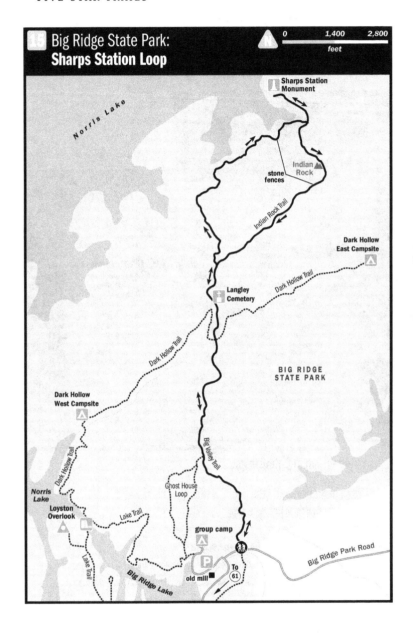

Big Ridge State Park:
Sharps Station Loop

Overview

Tread the back reaches of Big Ridge State Park on this trek. Follow old settler roads on the Big Valley Trail, topping Pinnacle Ridge. Pass the Langley Cemetery before scaling Big Ridge. From there, drop steeply to the shores of Norris Lake, where you visit a monument commemorating one of the first settlements west of the Appalachians. Your return route leads steeply up Big Ridge and past Indian Rock, with a winter view. Cruise a high bluff before backtracking to the trailhead.

Route Details

Your destination on this hike—Sharps Station—was one of the first white settlements west of the Appalachian Mountains. What was to be Knoxville, then known as Whites Fort, was the other. Nowadays, Knoxville is a thriving metropolis, while Sharps Station no longer exists. However, a plaque commemorates the location of Sharps Station, and you can walk to the site.

Note: Indian Rock Trail can be difficult to follow during the warm season, as it is lesser used and may be somewhat overgrown. Check with the park office about trail conditions if you are inexperienced.

Join Big Valley Trail, tracing a roadbed used by pre–Norris Dam settlers as an access to the Norton Gristmill, located near the

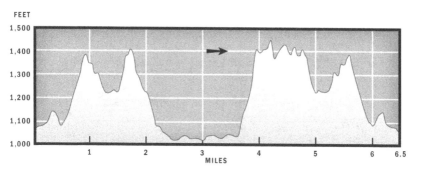

parking area. The forest is sparse in spots, recovering from a past attack by pine beetles, which downed many big evergreens. The trees are growing back but aren't yet high enough to produce shade. Top a hill at 0.3 miles, then dip to a narrow hollow. Bridge a streamlet at 0.5 miles, then climb a gullied track to meet the Ghost House Loop at 0.6 miles. Keep straight on Big Valley Trail, topping Pinnacle Ridge at 0.9 miles. Drift down to meet the Dark Hollow Trail at 1.3 miles.

Leave north from the intersection with the Dark Hollow Trail, climbing from a gap. Reach the Langley Cemetery at 1.6 miles, located on the narrow ridgeline. Most of the graves are simple, unmarked stones. The trail steepens while ascending the south slope of Big Ridge. Top out, catching your breath, then glide downhill, reaching a trail junction at 1.8 miles. Here, the loop portion of Indian Rock Trail splits. Stay left, now on a faint singletrack path diving toward Norris Lake, visible through the trees. Watch for paint blazes and flagging tape to help steer your course. The slope eases in mixed woods, formerly farmland. Turn northeasterly in flats. Step across a stony streambed at 2.2 miles, then turn left along it to meet the lakeshore near an embayment at 2.3 miles. Cruise parallel to the shore, coming to a second embayment. Find a forgotten stone fence, situated along a creek bed, at 2.8 miles. Continue through a cedar grove to reach a trail junction at 3 miles. The next streambed is just ahead. Here, Indian Rock Trail heads right and uphill and is your return route. To reach Sharps Station, stay left on Sharps Station Trail, crossing the rocky streambed and cruising along a limestone bluff before descending to another streambed. You are in piney flats, keeping the shoreline to your left. The path leads to a lakeside stone marker and nearly obscured gravestones at 3.3 miles. The fort located here provided protection from Indians for the intrepid settlers. The plaque, erected in 1967, mentions a particular December 1794 Indian attack. It is worthwhile to ponder what other events transpired that ultimately led to the abandonment of Sharps Station versus the expansion of Knoxville. Of course, the final blow to Sharps Station was the development of Norris Lake, which led to the displacement of many East Tennessee residents along what was then the free-flowing Clinch River.

Backtrack 0.3 miles from the plaque, enjoying a few lake views. Prepare for a challenging climb up a rib ridge, where you gain nearly 400 feet in 0.3 miles. The ascent eases at an outcrop known as Indian Rock. Here, an early settler named Peter Graves was ambushed and scalped by the natives. Graves was turkey hunting. While following the gobbles of a turkey he walked right to the Indians, who were really making the bird sounds from behind the rock outcrop you see.

The path tops out on Big Ridge, then turns southwest, running along an upturned rock spine shaded by tall trees. Pass a stone fence atop the bluffline at 4 miles. Drop to a gap at 4.2 miles. Undulate along the rocky ridgeline, then complete the loop portion of the hike at 4.7 miles. From here, backtrack 1.8 miles to the trailhead.

Nearby Attractions

The state park offers fishing, boating, and camping, in addition to hiking.

Directions

From Knoxville, take TN 33 north to TN 61. Follow TN 61 west 6.3 miles as it winds through hills to reach the state park on your right. Enter the park and drive a short distance to reach the old entrance station. The park office is to your left and offers maps. Keep straight beyond the station, passing the park cabins. After 0.6 miles reach a stop sign. Turn left here, parking near the Norton Gristmill replica. The trailhead is 0.2 miles east from the mill. Backtrack to the stop sign and walk a bit farther to reach Big Valley Trail, on the north side of the road.

Cumberland Trail above LaFollette

SCENERY: ★ ★ ★ ★ ★
TRAIL CONDITION: ★ ★
CHILDREN: ★
DIFFICULTY: ★ ★ ★
SOLITUDE: ★ ★ ★

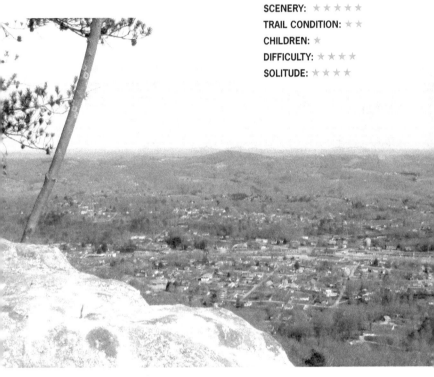

THE CUMBERLAND TRAIL IS TENNESSEE'S MASTER PATH.

GPS TRAILHEAD COORDINATES: N36° 23.284' W84° 7.550'

DISTANCE & CONFIGURATION: 5.6-mile out-and-back

HIKING TIME: 3.8 hours

HIGHLIGHTS: Spectacular ridgeline views, knife-edge rocks

ELEVATION: 1,100 feet at trailhead to 2,000 feet at high point

ACCESS: No fees, permits, or passes required; open year-round 24/7

MAPS: Cumberland Mountain segment of the Cumberland Trail, USGS Nydell, Jacksboro

FACILITIES: Trailhead spring

WHEELCHAIR ACCESS: None

CONTACTS: Cumberland Trail Conference, 19 East 4th St., Crossville, TN 38555; (931) 456-6259; **cumberlandtrail.org**

Overview

This is one spectacular hike. Follow the Cumberland Trail as it leaves the town of LaFollette, then climbs the slope of Cumberland Mountain. You will join a knife-edge ridge with protruding spinelike outcrops that offer expansive vistas. Peer upon LaFollette below and gaze southward to the Smoky Mountains and westward into the wild Cumberland Plateau, culminating in the Powell Valley Overlook. Beyond this vista, you'll encounter a backcountry trail shelter, a high-elevation stream, and Window Rock, a stone wall with a porthole in it.

Route Details

Big Creek Gap, where this hike begins, is the next major break in Cumberland Mountain south of Cumberland Gap, made famous by Daniel Boone and the Wilderness Road. Thirty miles south of Cumberland Gap, Big Creek Gap made a little history itself. During the Civil War, the gap was much narrower than it is now, before being widened to allow a road and railway to pass through. Confederate soldiers were stationed above the gap, and it became the site of an 1862 skirmish in which the Rebels were supplanted from their defensive position by the Yankees.

Nowadays, Tank Springs, located at the trailhead, attracts locals to the gap. If you hang around long enough you will see area residents filling jugs and taking the mountain water to their homes for drinking. Cumberland Trail (CT) trekkers can fill their bottles before making the nearly thousand-foot ascent to the high point of the hike. Be apprised the trail runs through the North Cumberland Wildlife Management Area; you can check for infrequent hunting dates via the Tennessee Wildlife Resources Agency website.

Pick up the wide-track path at Tank Springs by walking around a pole gate and passing a trailhead kiosk. Big Creek continues its work, cutting through the gap to your right, and US 25W rumbles with cars and trucks. A railroad line runs to your left. Altogether,

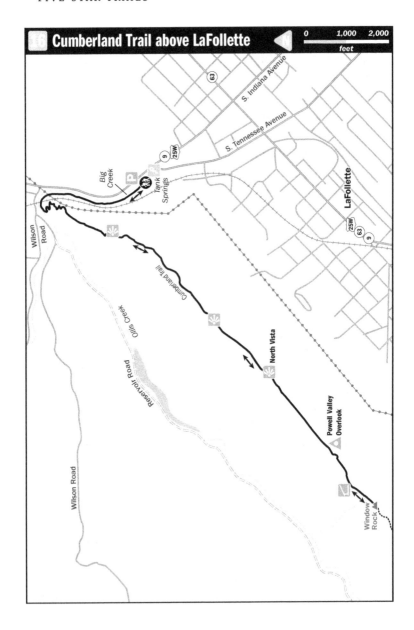

Cumberland Trail above LaFollette

0   1,000   2,000
feet

S. Indiana Avenue

63

S. Tennessee Avenue

9   25W

Big Creek

Tank Springs

LaFollette

25W
63   9

Wilson Road

Ollis Creek

Cumberland Trail

North Vista

Reservoir Road

Powell Valley Overlook

Wilson Road

Window Rock

you have railroad lines, automobiles, and hikers utilizing the gap, demonstrating its continued importance as a travel corridor.

Big Creek tumbles over rocks large and small, creating rapids and pools. An impressive rock promontory juts forth from the forest across the gap. You will soon be higher than that. But after a half mile the trail hasn't climbed a bit, and you begin to wonder if you have lost the trail, which travels under a railroad trestle spanning Ollis Creek just above its confluence with Big Creek. Beyond the trestle the Cumberland Trail turns sharply left and begins its ascent of Cumberland Mountain, using multiple switchbacks under a hardwood forest of maple, hickory, oak, and magnolia. At 0.7 miles, reach the foundation of a forgotten concrete structure.

Continue climbing as the ridgeline narrows and a rocky spine protrudes from the soil. Lichens, ferns, and mountain laurel border the path. At 1 mile, the steep pathway levels off, and you gain obscured views of LaFollette below and mountains to the north. Serviceberry trees grow among the outcrops. The CT then curves around the north side of a steep stone promontory, shortly regaining the crest of the ridge. At 1.1 miles, your first unobscured view opens up to the south, through Big Creek Gap. The crest of Cumberland Mountain briefly widens, then narrows and becomes rocky again. Keep climbing; you will reach the 1,800-foot elevation mark at 1.3 miles. A brief

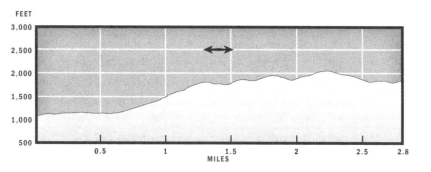

downgrade is welcome as you slip around the north side of a rock protrusion to make a shallow gap at 1.5 miles.

The white-blazed CT ascends from the gap on a rock spine, bordered by pines and mountain laurel, while galax hugs the forest floor. Work your way up the ragged, jagged crest that resembles upturned shark fins, with a serious drop-off below. Your next major vista opens at 1.7 miles. Here, LaFollette lies 800 feet beneath you. The Powell River Valley extends easterly. On a clear day Mount LeConte in the Smokies is easily identifiable. Buzzards may be floating the nearby thermals.

Dip to another gap at 2 miles. Climb away on another rock spine. Watch for a vista to the north at 2.1 miles. The contrast is amazing: Cumberland Mountain divides the civilized Powell River Valley from the scantly populated torturous terrain to the north. Reach your high point of 2,000 feet at 2.2 miles. The trail levels off, and you're walking atop rock slabs bordered by tightly grown young pines.

The views come fast and furious here. Note that the parallel rock ridge to your right, together with the outcrop you are walking, forms an elevated valley. At 2.6 miles, on a descent, the trail appears to end at an outcrop. You have reached the Powell Valley Overlook. Not only can you look south and east into the Powell River watershed but also west into the Catoosa Wildlife Management Area through which the Cumberland Trail travels. Less adventurous hikers may want to turn around here, but those not afraid of a little rock scrambling on all fours will work their way down the sandstone ledge (it's not far) before continuing southwesterly using only leg power to shortly reach a gap. At 2.8 miles, the CT climbs to a wooden trail shelter and campsite, located in a forested flat beside rock outcrops. Continue past the shelter and dip to a streamlet cloaked in rhododendron. A rock rampart rises beyond the watercourse. The CT travels along the rampart in a rich wildflower area. Look for Window Rock, an opening in the rock wall, in this little vale. Beyond here the CT continues southwesterly atop Cumberland Mountain to reach I-75 and Cove Lake State Park in 9 miles. After hiking here, you may want to support Tennessee's master path, the Cumberland Trail. Visit its website listed on page 100.

Directions

From Knoxville, take I-75 north to Exit 134, for Justin P. Wilson Cumberland Trail State Park. Take US 25W north 8.2 miles to LaFollette and turn left at traffic light #9 (the traffic lights are numbered), Indiana Avenue. Follow Indiana Avenue north 0.4 miles to a signed left turn for Justin P. Wilson Cumberland Trail State Park at Tennessee Street and cross Big Creek. Turn right into a parking area immediately after crossing Big Creek.

17 Devils Backbone

SCENERY: ★ ★ ★ ★
TRAIL CONDITION: ★ ★
CHILDREN: ★ ★
DIFFICULTY: ★ ★ ★
SOLITUDE: ★ ★ ★ ★

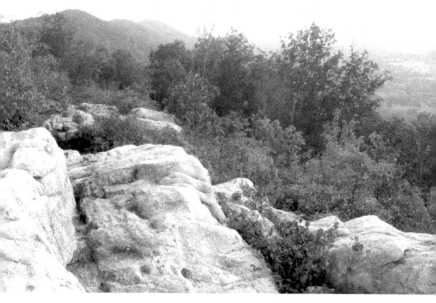

GREAT VIEWS AWAIT THOSE WHO CLIMB DEVILS BACKBONE.

GPS TRAILHEAD COORDINATES: N36° 18.441' W84° 13.625'
DISTANCE & CONFIGURATION: 6-mile out-and-back
HIKING TIME: 3.4 hours
HIGHLIGHTS: Waterfalls, rock outcrops, wide views
ELEVATION: 1,050 feet at trailhead to 1,830 feet at high point
ACCESS: No fees, permits, or passes required; open year-round 24/7
MAPS: Cumberland Mountain segment of Cumberland Trail, USGS Jacksboro
FACILITIES: None
WHEELCHAIR ACCESS: None
CONTACTS: Cumberland Trail Conference, 19 East 4th St., Crossville, TN 38555; (931) 456-6259; **cumberlandtrail.org**

Overview

This hike uses the Cumberland Trail to reach a spectacular view from the rocky western edge of Cumberland Mountain, known as Devils Backbone. Along the way you will pass some steep falls. Be apprised the trail travels very near I-75, so you will be exposed to road noise. However, the highlights are worth it.

Route Details

Just about everyone who drives north up I-75 from Knoxville notices Devils Backbone. The backbone is a series of upturned exposed rock "fins" that rise from the surrounding forest up the crest of Cumberland Mountain. It is only natural that a segment of the Cumberland Trail (CT) would travel to this distinct feature. Once you make it to Devils Backbone, your efforts will be well rewarded with far-reaching views to the south of the Clinch River Valley, much of which is dammed up as Norris Lake. To your west lies an endless series of ridges of the Cumberland Mountains, and you can clearly see the road outline of I-75 as it leads toward Knoxville. Speaking of I-75, it will be your nearly constant companion as you travel from the outreaches of Cove Lake State Park north to Devils Backbone. And yes, it is irritating. That said, I still recommend the hike. Others will second the motion; the trek to Devils Backbone is increasing in popularity, as is the entire Cumberland Trail.

Leave the Cumberland Trail parking area on a gravel path. Cove Creek flows to your left. The auto noise of I-75 swirls in the air, but don't sweat it. Pass a trailside kiosk and keep straight to meet a trail junction. Here, the Smoky Mountain segment of the Cumberland Trail splits left, aiming for Frozen Head State Park. Stay right on a singletrack path that rises by switchbacks. Rich woods with scattered large oaks offer visual beauty. Pass through an old burn with more scrubby woods. After 0.3 miles, reach another trail junction. Here, the Volunteer Loop leads right. You can use it for your return route. The Cumberland Trail keeps its northerly direction. In winter, you will

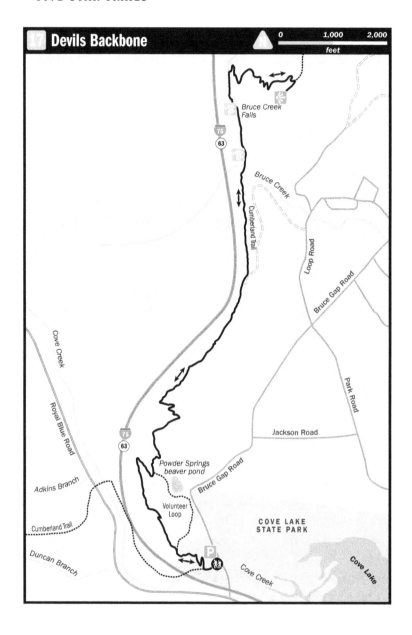

Devils Backbone

0   1,000   2,000
feet

Bruce Creek
Falls

75
63

Bruce Creek

Cumberland Trail

Loop Road

Bruce Gap Road

Cove Creek

Park Road

Royal Blue Road

75
63

Jackson Road

Adkins Branch

Powder Springs
beaver pond

Bruce Gap Road

Cumberland Trail

Volunteer
Loop

COVE LAKE
STATE PARK

Duncan Branch

P

Cove Creek

Cove Lake

see Cumberland Mountain rising above. Pass a huge oak just before reaching the other end of the Volunteer Loop at 0.8 miles. Descend to a sycamore-laden flat, then ascend along a trickling branch. The CT switchbacks away from the streamlet into a cedar-shaded rock field.

Reach a gap at 1.3 miles. The interstate is just to your left. The CT bridges a giant gully at 1.4 miles, then surmounts a fence at 1.6 miles. You are practically close enough to the interstate to feel a breeze from the trucks going by. Bisect brushy woods that can be overgrown in summer. Views open to the east. Enter a boulder field at 2 miles. This boulder field is clearly not natural. The rocks were sent down the hillside when the interstate was built. The trail opens onto a talus slope, then dips to meet Bruce Creek at an old road at 2.1 miles. Stay left here. Bruce Creek tumbles in the numerous waterfalls. Yet a closer examination will reveal that the watercourse was rerouted with the building of the interstate. The streambed is not natural and neither are the falls; the engineers had to work the water down and thus created the falls.

Continue walking through the scenic valley, which shields road noise. Pass a couple of campsites, reaching Bruce Falls at 2.3 miles. Clear water drops in four tiers into surprisingly deep pools. At 2.5 miles, bridge Bruce Creek. Begin switchbacking toward the crest of Cumberland Mountain, partially shaded by pines. Briefly level off in a flat before resuming the climb. Pass a huge erratic boulder that

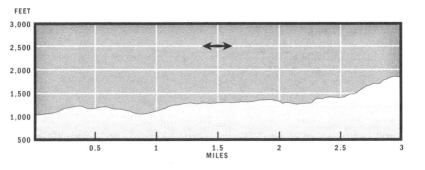

tumbled down from the crest of Cumberland Mountain to rest here in the woods. Avoid shortcutting the switchbacks. The building and maintenance of the Cumberland Trail is a volunteer project, so when shortcutting the switchbacks you cause erosion and mitigate the labor of people who are keeping Tennessee's master path in shape.

The sometimes-sandy trail bed tops out on Cumberland Mountain at 2.9 miles. Turn right here, leaving the CT, as it heads northeast to end at Cumberland Gap National Park. Travel a rocky track pocked with low-slung trees. Continue in pure rock to reach the tip of Devils Backbone at 3 miles. Your trail companion, I-75, is visible below. Southward, you can see Jacksboro in the immediate foreground and greater Knoxville and the crest of the Appalachians in the distance. Easterly, Cumberland Mountain undulates to the horizon. Westerly, the bulk of the Cumberland Plateau rises as a dark, wild rampart. Wow! On your return 3-mile trip, consider taking the Volunteer Loop. It cruises by Powder Springs beaver pond, then meanders low hills before rejoining the CT.

Nearby Attractions

Cove Lake State Park has a network of paved trails, a lake for fishing, and camping.

Directions

From Knoxville, take I-75 north to Exit 134. After exiting the interstate, turn left, crossing over to the west side of I-75 and away from Cove Lake State Park, on Old Highway 63. Follow Old Highway 63 past the Caryville municipal building for a total of 0.7 miles to Bruce Gap Road. Turn right on Bruce Gap Road and follow it back under the interstate 0.1 mile to the Cumberland Trail parking area on your left.

Norris Dam State Park:
Andrews Ridge Loop

SCENERY: ★ ★ ★
TRAIL CONDITION: ★ ★ ★ ★ ★
CHILDREN: ★ ★ ★
DIFFICULTY: ★ ★
SOLITUDE: ★ ★ ★ ★

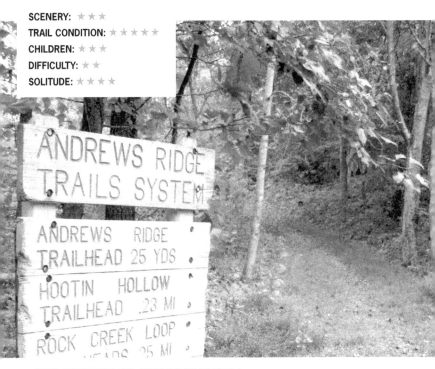

YOUR GATEWAY TO THE ANDREWS RIDGE TRAILS

GPS TRAILHEAD COORDINATES: N36° 14.506' W84° 7.445'

DISTANCE & CONFIGURATION: 4.7-mile triple loop

HIKING TIME: 2.5 hours

HIGHLIGHTS: Historic homesites, lake views

ELEVATION: 1,340 feet at trailhead to 1,050 feet at low point

ACCESS: No fees, permits, or passes required; open 8 a.m.–sunset

MAPS: Norris Dam State Park Trails, USGS Norris, Lake City, Demory, Jacksboro

FACILITIES: Restrooms, water at nearby campground

WHEELCHAIR ACCESS: None

CONTACTS: Norris Dam State Park, 125 Village Green Circle, Lake City, TN 37769; (865) 426-7461; **tnstateparks.com**

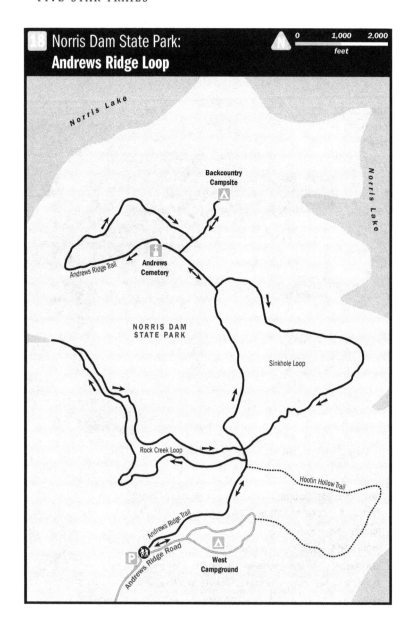

18 Norris Dam State Park:
Andrews Ridge Loop

0   1,000   2,000
feet

Norris Lake

Norris Lake

Backcountry
Campsite

Andrews Ridge Trail

Andrews
Cemetery

NORRIS DAM
STATE PARK

Sinkhole Loop

Rock Creek Loop

Hootin Hollow Trail

Andrews Ridge Trail

Andrews Ridge Road

West
Campground

Overview

This hike explores a distinct trail system at Norris Dam State Park. It follows old pioneer roads in hills and hollows homesteaded by rural Tennesseans displaced after the development of Norris Lake. Visit a quiet ridgetop cemetery between loops along steeply sloped ground.

Route Details

Andrews Ridge is bordered on three sides by the Cove Creek arm of Norris Lake. The dry hilltop was once home to settlers who labored on its hillsides, scratching out a subsistence living on hardscrabble farms and collecting drinking water from rooftop cisterns. So when word came that the Norris Lake project was going to require them to sell their land, it gave them an opportunity for a new start. Despite the land's less-than-ideal productivity, some people didn't want to move but were forced to. Now Andrews Ridge is part of Norris Dam State Park.

Over the ensuing generations, Andrews Ridge has reverted from field to woodland. The trails you follow trace mostly pioneer roads, weaving around the hills and hollows of the land. I wonder what the former residents would think if they came back to see their land as a recreation destination, with a modern campground and trails. You start this hike near the West Campground's RV dump station, tracing

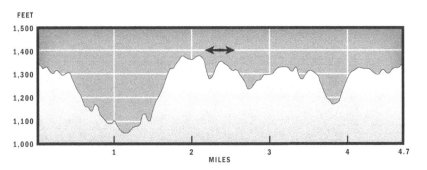

Andrews Ridge Trail, an old doubletrack road, heading north. Begin to look for artifacts such as old bricks, relics of past settlement. Beech, maple, pine, and tulip trees grow tall on the once-tilled hillsides.

At 0.4 miles, the Hootin Hollow Trail leaves right, curving into an embayment before ending at the West Campground. Keep straight on Andrews Ridge Trail and shortly meet Rock Creek Loop. It leads left and downhill, making a loop of its own. Dive into a hollow on the Rock Creek Loop. Look for old roads spurring off the main trail, though the way is clear. Bridge a wet-weather tributary and resume your descent toward Norris Lake. Wooded hills rise sharply around you, cut by streambeds flowing off Andrews Ridge. At 1 mile, reach a junction. Note the old-growth gray-trunked beech tree here. Continue down the hollow, now dominated by sycamores and buckeyes, crossing the main streambed three times to reach the shores of Norris Lake at 1.2 miles. If the water is down, an exposed mud bottom may separate you from the lake. Be careful along the shore or you may find yourself knee-deep in muck.

Begin backtracking away from the lake, rising into drier forests of oak and hickory to reach Andrews Ridge at 1.8 miles. Turn left, heading farther north on the Andrews Ridge Trail. Dogwood, black gum, sassafras, and sourwood flank the undulating path. Pass the north end of the Sinkhole Trail at 2.2 miles. At 2.3 miles, reach the loop portion of the Andrews Ridge Trail and stay left, shortly passing the small Andrews Cemetery. Here, lonely graves stand on a high point reclaimed by the forest and creeping periwinkle. Lake views open to the west beyond the cemetery. Meet the spur trail to the park's backcountry campsite at 3.1 miles. Follow it to dead-end at a fire ring and level spot. Overnight hikers must register at the park office and bring their own drinking water to this camp. Complete the loop on Andrews Ridge at 3.4 miles after backtracking from the campsite.

Begin your final circuit at 3.5 miles, turning left on the Sinkhole Loop. This trail curves along the easterly slope of Andrews Ridge, descending to a gap at 3.6 miles, then resumes following the contours of the lake below. At 4.3 miles, complete the Sinkhole

Loop. From here, backtrack 0.4 miles to the trailhead. If you want to extend your hike, take the Hootin Hollow Trail 0.7 miles to reach the West Campground, then follow the campground access road to the trailhead.

Nearby Attractions

Norris Dam has recreation opportunities aplenty in addition to trails. Overnight in a cabin, go boating on Norris Lake, or camp in one of two campgrounds to expand your hiking adventure.

Directions

From Exit 128 (Lake City) on I-75, take US 441 south 2.8 miles to the entrance of Norris Dam State Park. Turn left into the entrance and drive 0.3 miles to a road split. Head left for the West Campground and hiking trails. Drive 1.3 miles to the campground entrance station across from an RV dump station. There are several parking spots here. Please do not block the dump-station road.

19

Norris Dam State Park:
Lake View Trail

SCENERY: ★ ★ ★
TRAIL CONDITION: ★ ★ ★ ★
CHILDREN: ★ ★ ★
DIFFICULTY: ★ ★
SOLITUDE: ★ ★ ★

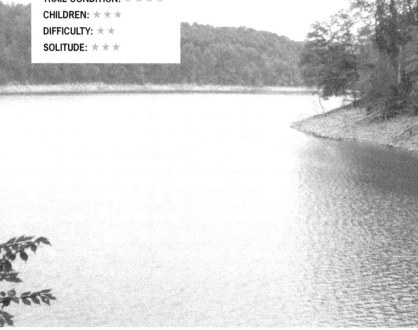

THE RICHLY WOODED SHORELINE OF NORRIS LAKE

GPS TRAILHEAD COORDINATES: N36° 13.566' W84° 5.326'

DISTANCE & CONFIGURATION: 3.6-mile triple loop

HIKING TIME: 2 hours

HIGHLIGHTS: Lake views, big trees

ELEVATION: 1,070 feet at trailhead to 1,450 feet at high point

ACCESS: No fees, passes, or permits required; open 8 a.m.–sunset

MAPS: Norris Dam State Park Trails, USGS Norris

FACILITIES: Restrooms, water, and picnic area at state park and nearby dam visitor center

WHEELCHAIR ACCESS: None

CONTACTS: Norris Dam State Park, 125 Village Green Circle, Lake City, TN 37769;
(865) 426-7461; **tnstateparks.com**

Overview

This hike combines trails old and new. Start at Norris Dam on a Civilian Conservation Corps–built track along Norris Lake, traveling a steep slope with big trees. Then pick up the newer Lake View Trail, which explores more shoreline, with expansive water vistas, everywhere-you-look beauty, and still more big trees.

Route Details

This hike wanders a north-facing slope overlooking the lowermost part of Norris Lake, near Norris Dam, and features views many big trees along the way. Rich woods of beech tower overhead as you travel the hillside, running roughly parallel with the shoreline. Pass High Point on the return trip before joining nature trails that return you to Norris Dam. You will have to negotiate many trail junctions, but the way is clear and navigable by anyone.

The trek begins on a hiker-only asphalt path, Lakeside Loop Trail, leaving from big Norris Dam. The trail shortly changes to gravel. An angler's trail spurs left toward the shore, while the main track makes an easterly course under shade-bearing beeches. The still waters of Norris Lake are visible through the trees no matter the season. After a quarter mile the trail splits. Stay left, closer to the lake. At 0.3 miles, some old steps lead down to the lake, an earlier recreational incarnation of Norris Dam State Park. It looks like part of an old dock. This state park was originally developed in the 1930s. Over nine decades it has undergone many changes and displayed several recreational faces for visitors. The first of many clear lake views opens at this locale.

Continue on the moist north slope and shortly reach another junction. Here, Christmas Fern Trail leads right and uphill, but you stay left, joining Tall Timbers Trail. Begin curving around a cove of the lake under sycamore and tulip trees, making a mostly level track. Repose benches are set along the path, should you choose to relax. Meet the other end of Christmas Fern Trail at 0.5 miles. Keep

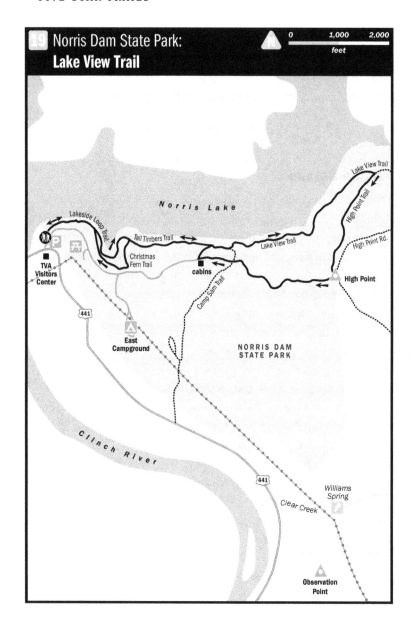

19 Norris Dam State Park:
Lake View Trail

0   1,000   2,000
feet

Lake View Trail

High Point Trail

N o r r i s   L a k e

Lakeside Loop Trail

Tall Timbers Trail

Lake View Trail

High Point Rd.

Christmas
Fern Trail

TVA
Visitors
Center

cabins

Camp Sam Trail

High Point

441

East
Campground

NORRIS DAM
STATE PARK

C l i n c h   R i v e r

441

Williams
Spring

Clear Creek

Observation
Point

straight on Tall Timbers Trail, still within the original state park trail system, built so long ago.

At 0.9 miles, you leave the older trail system and join the newer, multiuse Lake View Trail. This path was constructed in 2009 and ties together trails of the state park along with the City of Norris Watershed Trails, even though Lake View Trail stays within the bounds of the state park. Pass a horse barrier, then reach yet another split. Stay left as a sign warns equestrians to walk their horses on the super-steep gravelly track. Lunge toward Norris Lake.

Continue easterly in oak woods, also looking for impressive-sized buckeye and beech trees, including a huge old-growth beech at 1.3 miles on trail right. You'll experience more vertical variation in this section. Cove Creek Wildlife Management Area stands across the lake and provides a natural shoreline vista across the dammed waters of the Clinch River.

At 1.6 miles, meet the High Point Spur, which cuts back acutely right and uphill. Take this trail as it climbs through huge oak trees to reach High Point at 2.1 miles, a wooded spot (no views) and trail intersection. You are nearly 400 feet higher than when you started. A trailside kiosk helps keep hikers oriented. Turn right here, now heading westerly on a doubletrack trail. Short spurs dead-end—just stay with the well-trod path.

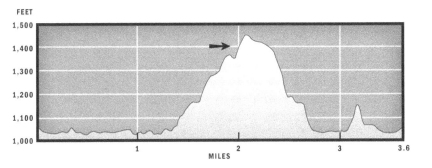

At 2.3 miles, the path angles right and downhill, passing around a chain-link gate. Keep descending under more big oaks to reach a four-way trail junction at 2.5 miles. Here, Camp Sam Trail leads left and a spur trail leads right back toward the Lake View Trail. This hike keeps forward to pass around a gate and reach a park cabin cluster. Pass Cabin #10 on your left, then look for a slender trail leading right, away from the cabins, at 2.6 miles.

Begin backtracking at 2.7 miles, again in the network of old nature trails, heading west along Tall Timbers Trail. Enjoy some new terrain as you pick up the Christmas Fern Trail leading left and uphill at 3.1 miles. Ascend through paw paws, nearing a park road before dropping to another intersection at 3.3 miles. Keep left on Lakeview Loop Trail before returning to the trailhead at 3.6 miles.

Nearby Attractions

Norris Dam has recreation opportunities aplenty in addition to trails. Overnight in a cabin, go boating on Norris Lake, or camp in one of two campgrounds to expand your hiking adventure.

Directions

From Knoxville, take I-75 north to Exit 122. Turn right on TN 61 east and follow it 1.4 miles to US 441. Turn left and take US 441 north 4.9 miles, passing the TVA visitors center on your left just before reaching Norris Dam State Park East Area. Park in the circular lot on the right just before US 441 crosses Norris Dam.

20

Norris Dam State Park:
Marine Railway Loop

SCENERY: ★ ★ ★
TRAIL CONDITION: ★ ★ ★ ★
CHILDREN: ★ ★ ★
DIFFICULTY: ★ ★ ★
SOLITUDE: ★ ★ ★

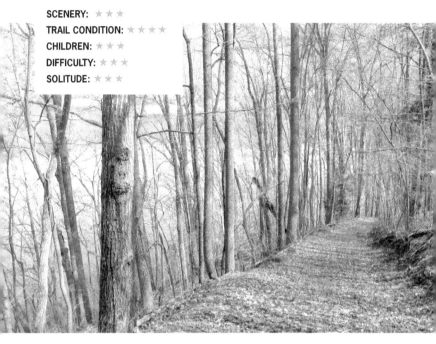

WINTER VIEW OF NORRIS LAKE

GPS TRAILHEAD COORDINATES: N36° 14.598 W84° 6.132

DISTANCE & CONFIGURATION: 3.5-mile double loop

HIKING TIME: 2 hours

HIGHLIGHTS: Lake views, wide trail

ELEVATION: 1,310 feet at trailhead to 1,050 feet at low point

ACCESS: No fees, permits, or passes required; open 8 a.m.–sunset

MAPS: Norris Dam State Park Trails, USGS Norris

FACILITIES: Restrooms, water, picnic, playground, campground at state park

WHEELCHAIR ACCESS: None

COMMENTS: Cabins at trailhead

CONTACTS: Norris Dam State Park, 125 Village Green Circle, Lake City, TN 37769; (865) 426-7461; **tnstateparks.com**

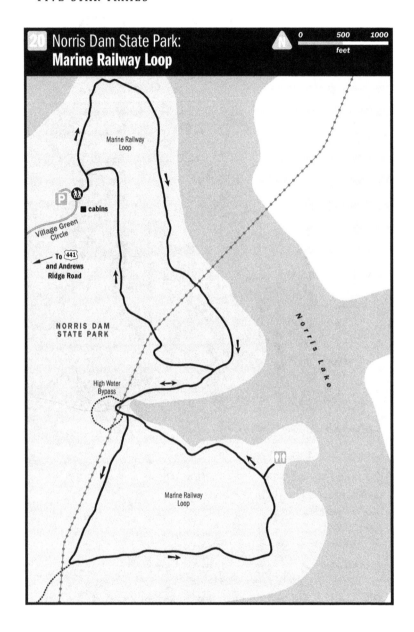

20 Norris Dam State Park:
Marine Railway Loop

0   500   1000
feet

Marine Railway
Loop

P

cabins

Village Green
Circle

To 441
and Andrews
Ridge Road

NORRIS DAM
STATE PARK

High Water
Bypass

Norris Lake

Marine Railway
Loop

Overview

This doubletrack path located at Norris Dam State Park starts atop a knobby ridge before plunging toward Norris Lake, where it travels near the shore through second-growth forest. The hike then turns up an inlet, where it makes a second loop and climbs the knobby ridge again, only to return to Norris Lake, this time passing directly along accessible shoreline. Your second climb, back to the trailhead, is gentler. Norris Dam State Park offers many other trails as well as other recreational opportunities.

Route Details

Norris Dam State Park is chock-full of trails. The Marine Railway Loop is but one hiking opportunity, but trail treaders seem to gravitate to this path because so much of it goes along scenic Norris Lake. What started as a flood-control project—Norris Dam—begun during the Great Depression has resulted in this park with lake, river, and land recreation administered by the state of Tennessee and the Tennessee Valley Authority, more commonly referred to as TVA.

 The hike makes somewhat of an odd start, as you have to walk behind Cabin #8, a state park rental cabin that may be occupied. But don't sweat it; pick up the wide trail leading downhill and left away from Cabin #8. Shortly reach a signed trail intersection and

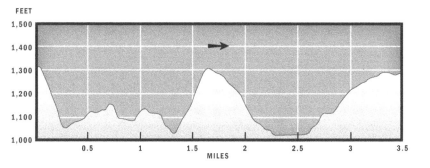

the beginning of the actual Marine Railway Loop. Turn left here, northerly, heading sharply downhill on a shaded doubletrack path that makes walking easy and allows you to enjoy the surrounding woodland environs. In winter you will already be viewing Norris Lake as it nearly encircles the peninsula down which you hike.

Chestnut oak, red oak, maple, and other hardwoods shade the path as it dives for the water. Norris Lake is quite serpentine. The dammed waters of the Clinch River and Powell River both cut torturous courses through the knobby ridges forming the transition between the Cumberland Plateau and the Tennessee River Valley. It is this relationship between water and land that makes Norris Lake one of the most scenic bodies of water in the South.

Level off after 0.25 miles, then curve easterly. The impoundment, with all its fingerlike inlets, lies to your left. You are actually on the Cove Creek Arm of the lake. Red maple, tulip, dogwood, and beech trees find their niche in the forest, while pine, cedar, and the occasional hemlock add year-round greenery. Pass under a power line cut at 0.8 miles. Of course, having a power line so near the electricity-generating Norris Dam should be no surprise. The clear-cut offers an unobstructed vantage of Norris Lake. At 0.9 miles, turn into a narrow bay. Reach a trail junction at 1 mile. Your return route and the first loop leave to the right, but you stay left, heading for the second loop along the narrow bay.

The trail descends toward the top of the inlet. Watch as the High Water Bypass leaves to the right. Use the bypass when Norris Lake is up and floods the main trail; otherwise, curve around the inlet, ignoring a closed power line access road at the inlet head. Reach a trail junction at 1.3 miles. Here, the other end of the High Water Bypass enters, and just ahead the second loop begins. Turn right here, southerly, aiming up the hill under the power line. It's an ugly steep climb, and you can see every bit of elevation to be gained. Numerically speaking, it is 280 feet in 0.3 miles, where you reach a trail junction. The trail leading right, still southerly, meets US 441 and is an alternate trailhead for the Marine Railway Loop. This hike, however, leads acutely left, easterly, toward Norris Lake.

The downgrade is shaded by hardwoods and is gentler than the climb you just made, descending the same distance climbed in 0.5 miles. Norris Dam is visible through the trees to the south. Drift into flatlands and reach a trail junction at 2.2 miles. Here, a spur trail leaves right to a bench overlooking a piney peninsula and a lake-access point where you could swim or play fetch with a water-loving dog. When the lake is at its drawn-down winter levels, you will see artificial fish attraction structures embedded in the lake bottom.

Resume the loop, curving along the inlet you were at before, this time directly along the shoreline. Note the numerous trees fallen into the lake's edge. They also provide good fish habitat. Reach a trail junction at 2.5 miles, completing the second loop. Backtrack around the inlet and reach the first loop at 2.8 miles. Stay left, northwesterly, making your second climb, which is fairly gradual. Pass under the power line a final time. Resume hiking under hardwoods, watching for redbuds and dogwoods. Complete the second loop. Cabin #8 is within sight through the trees. Backtrack to the trailhead to complete the 3.5-mile hike.

Other trails are nearby. The Andrews Ridge trail system is detailed in this guidebook on page 111. It leaves from the state park's West Campground. The Norris Watershed Trails, also known as the East Park Trail System, explores the terrain east of Norris Dam. TVA offers still more trails, including River Bluff Trail, detailed in this guidebook on page 132.

Nearby Attractions

Norris Dam has recreational opportunities aplenty in addition to trails. Overnight in a cabin, go boating on Norris Lake, or camp in one of two campgrounds to expand your hiking adventure.

Directions

From Exit 128 (Lake City) on I-75, take US 441 south 2.8 miles to the entrance of Norris Dam State Park. Turn left into the entrance and drive 0.3 miles to a road split. Stay right, heading toward the park office and park cabins. Pass the park office on your left. Stop and get a trail map. Continue toward the cabins; follow the paved road to its end in a cul-de-sac. Park here. To pick up the trail, walk a short distance back toward Cabin #8. The trail starts behind Cabin #8.

SCENERY: ★ ★ ★ ★
TRAIL CONDITION: ★ ★ ★ ★
CHILDREN: ★ ★ ★
DIFFICULTY: ★ ★
SOLITUDE: ★ ★

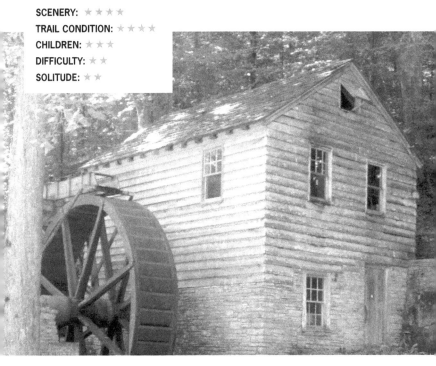

GRISTMILL BESIDE CLEAR CREEK

GPS TRAILHEAD COORDINATES: N36° 12.783' W84° 4.347'

DISTANCE & CONFIGURATION: 3.7-mile loop

HIKING TIME: 2 hours

HIGHLIGHTS: Historic gristmill, cleared vistas

ELEVATION: 880 feet at trailhead to 1,360 feet at high point

ACCESS: No fees, permits, or passes required; open dawn to dusk

MAPS: Norris Watershed Trail Map, USGS Norris

FACILITIES: Restrooms, water fountain, picnic tables at Norris Dam visitor center

WHEELCHAIR ACCESS: None

COMMENTS: This is but one hike in the extensive Norris Watershed trail system.

CONTACTS: City of Norris, 20 Chestnut Dr., P.O. Box 1090, Norris, TN 37828; (865) 494-7645; **cityofnorris.com**

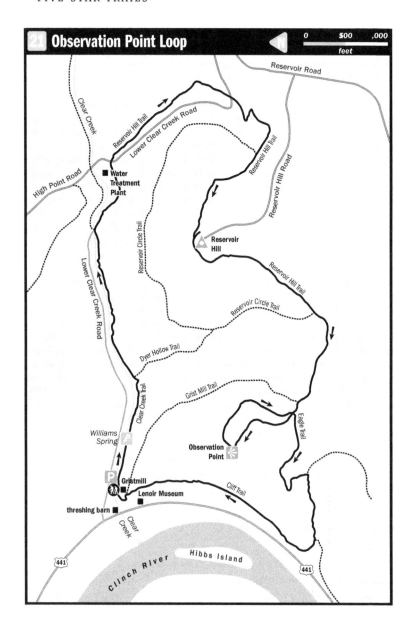

Overview

This is a great hike on land originally acquired by TVA as part of Norris Dam, on trails developed by the Civilian Conservation Corps in the 1930s. Begin on scenic Clear Creek at a historic gristmill. Travel along the cool valley of the stream before rising to a view atop Reservoir Hill. Travel through tall timber to Observation Point, a superlative clear overlook of the Clinch River Valley, Norris Dam, and Cumberland Mountain beyond. Descend along a steep riverside bluff to complete the loop.

Route Details

The Norris Watershed trails are located below Norris Dam. They offer well-marked and maintained singletrack and doubletrack paths winding through a surprisingly large area, especially when you combine it with the property of adjacent Norris Dam State Park. This particular hike travels along lower Clear Creek, a slender, crystalline stream broken by small dams. The path then leaves the stream and ascends into hickories and oaks on Reservoir Hill, site of a large water storage tank and a shaded picnic area with attractive stonework. Travel under some large trees that perhaps escaped the logger's axe before making a side trip to aptly named Observation Point, an overlook that accurately captures East Tennessee with its

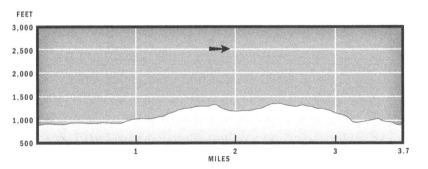

rivers, ridges, mountains, and lakes. It also captures the essence of the Tennessee Valley Authority, which shaped this land and its people as much as any other single influence.

The hike begins at the old gristmill. Explore the primitive power plant, parts of which have been in operation since 1798. The mill, originally constructed in nearby Union County, Tennessee, has undergone many changes and was moved to its present site; otherwise, it would have been flooded under Norris Lake, as so many other lifeways were. Follow Clear Creek Trail beyond the mill, joining a sluiceway that delivers water from Williams Spring to turn the mill wheel. Pass the springhead, emerging from the base of a tree. Travel under a pair of power line cuts, as a spur path goes to a streamside picnic area. Meet Dyer Hollow Trail at 0.3 miles. Keep straight on Clear Creek Trail, curving past some small stone dams on Clear Creek. The stream spills noisily over these dams. This was once the site of a now-vanished gristmill.

The cool, moist corridor is good for spring wildflowers. Reach Lower Clear Creek Road at 0.7 miles. Look across the road for the rectangular water runs from a small fish hatchery. Clear Creek Trail now wanders the far side of Clear Creek. You can take it or walk up the road to the Norris water treatment plant. Here, Hi Point Trail leaves left as a road across Clear Creek. This hike stays right, joining Reservoir Hill Trail as it turns south and runs parallel to Lower Clear Creek Road.

Ascend, crossing Lower Clear Creek Road at 1.2 miles. Keep climbing into oaks, passing a sinkhole before meeting Reservoir Circle Trail at 1.4 miles. More climbing, and you'll come to a decorative stone wall and shaded picnic area at 1.7 miles. Spur trails lead to the picnic area, where you can grab a view through the trees of Norris Dam. Head downhill among large, regal oaks. Intersect the other end of Reservoir Circle Trail at 2 miles. Keep straight, bisecting two power line clearings before meeting the Grist Mill Trail at 2.3 miles. It is just 0.7 miles to the parking area, but why cut short the hike when the best is yet to come?

Instead, keep straight, and in a few feet arrive at another junction. Here, take the teardrop Observation Point Trail. Loop up to a gazebo and Observation Point at 2.5 miles. Here, you can gaze northwest to soak in Norris Dam, the Clinch River flowing below, hills spreading off, and finally Cumberland Mountain rising in the background. What a sight! No wonder the CCC boys routed a trail here! Listen to the roar as the Clinch flows over the weir dam below.

Loop back down to the junction, then pick up the Eagle Trail, a slender singletrack path descending off the hill of Observation Point. Pass a dead-end trail leaving left at 3 miles, then continue descending a hollow to reach another intersection at 3.1 miles. A spur leads left down to US 441. Watch for a low-flow fall dripping over a stone lip just above this junction. This hike leaves right and uphill on the Cliff Trail. Curve onto a sharply sloped wooded bluff above the Clinch River. Look down on the river and weir dam. The slope eases and you meet the Grist Mill Trail just before coming to the Lenoir Museum. It is but a short walk to the trailhead from the museum to finish the 3.7-mile walk.

Nearby Attractions

Nearby Norris Dam State Park offers camping, picnicking, and more hiking. The Clinch River has first-rate trout fishing and paddling opportunities. Norris Lake offers flatwater boating and fishing.

Directions

From Knoxville, take I-75 north to Exit 122. Turn right on TN 61 east and follow it 1.4 miles to US 441. Turn left and take US 441 north 3.6 miles. Look for the right turn to Lower Clear Creek Road and a sign for the gristmill. This turn is just past the Lenoir Museum. Park by the old gristmill. If this lot is full, park at the Lenoir Museum.

River Bluff Trail

SCENERY: ★ ★ ★
TRAIL CONDITION: ★ ★ ★ ★
CHILDREN: ★ ★ ★ ★
DIFFICULTY: ★ ★
SOLITUDE: ★ ★ ★

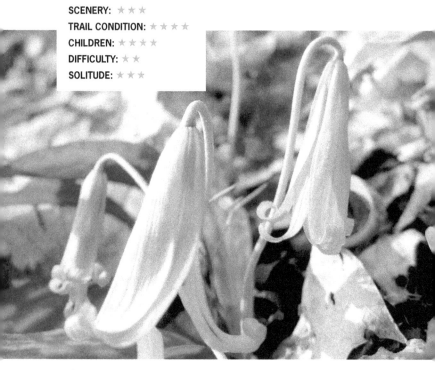

WILDFLOWERS ABOUND ON THIS TRAIL IN SPRING.

GPS TRAILHEAD COORDINATES: N36° 13.227' W84° 5.703'

DISTANCE & CONFIGURATION: 3.3-mile loop

HIKING TIME: 1.9 hours

HIGHLIGHTS: River views, spring wildflowers

ELEVATION: 820 feet at low point to 1,140 feet at high point

ACCESS: No fees, permits, or passes required; open 8 a.m.–dusk

MAPS: Norris Dam State Park, USGS Norris

FACILITIES: None

WHEELCHAIR ACCESS: None

COMMENTS: Many other trails are nearby on this TVA property and at Norris Dam State Park.

CONTACTS: Tennessee Valley Authority, 400 West Summit Hill Dr., Knoxville, TN 37902; (865) 632-2101; **tva.com**

Overview

The Tennessee Valley Authority (TVA) did a good job in locating a trail on this bluff below Norris Dam. The steep north-facing slope overlooks the Clinch River and offers superlative wildflower displays amid sheer rock outcrops and tall forest. It also provides a good workout after traveling downstream along the trout-filled tailwater when it climbs the bluff. The return trip meanders under oaks along the bluff edge, exploring multiple environments.

Route Details

Leave easterly from the parking area on a singletrack footpath. The federally designated national recreation trail travels beneath white oak, hickory, beech, and holly in a TVA-designated natural area. The moist, north-facing slope upon which it travels makes it nearly ideal for wildflowers in April. Among the spring offerings you will see are trillium, trout lily, mayapple, toothwort, and wild ginger. The path drifts closer to the Clinch River, which Norris Dam impounds as Norris Lake. The dam is located within sight of the trail. In winter you can easily see the concrete behemoth through the trees. The road you came in on once accessed the lower dam but is now gated for security. On a still day you will undoubtedly hear the hum of the dam as its turbines create electricity.

Norris Dam was TVA's first impoundment, completed in 1936. Many residents were unhappy about being removed from the fertile riverside lands for Norris Lake. TVA tried to make good relations by showing how the project would benefit the greater whole of society. One way they did this was making demonstration parks along the newly created lake and dam. The lands that the River Bluff Trail explores are part of the demonstration parks, as are nearby Norris Dam State Park and Big Ridge State Park, both of which feature hiking trails included in this guidebook.

Reach the loop portion of your hike at 0.3 miles. Stay left, still easterly, on the singletrack. Ferns and mosses also thrive on this north

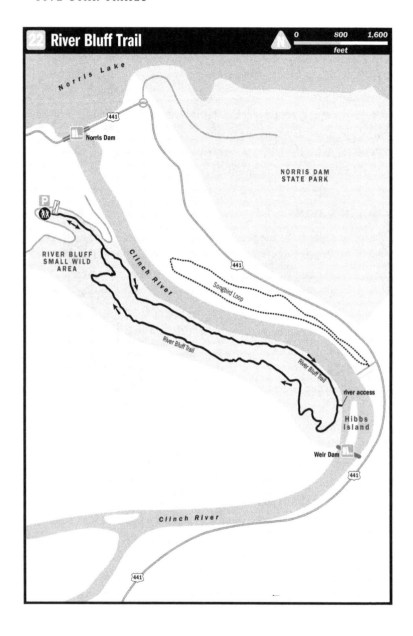

slope. Bridge a steep, wet-weather stream at 0.4 miles. Trout lilies seemingly cover the entire slope in this area during April. Come along the Clinch River at 0.7 miles. The clear green aqua is quite cold after emerging from the dam base. This icy water supports a trout fishery. In summer you may feel a cool breeze blowing off the water. Depending upon whether the dam is generating or not you may see anglers in waders or in boats fishing the river. Fallen trees line the water's edge and provide habitat for trout. On the land, mossy rock outcrops rise above you. Buckeye trees are quite common on this lower slope.

Thus far the elevation undulations have been negligible. Look uphill for a sheer bluff rising forth from the thick forest. The trail traces the river as the waterway turns southeasterly. At 1.4 miles, watch for a boat ramp across the river as well as trails. In winter you may even see hikers walking the Songbird Trail, an easy trek on level terrain. At 1.5 miles, come to a bench and a trail leading left to river access. Walk down and touch the chilly water as it divides around the head of Hibbs Island. A weir dam located at the base of Hibbs Island oxygenates the water, making it a better environment for fish and other aquatic species.

River Bluff Trail turns away from the water, making a pair of switchbacks as it heads for higher ground. The Clinch continues its journey, only to be impounded by Melton Hill Reservoir, then freed once again to meet the Tennessee River near the town of Kingston.

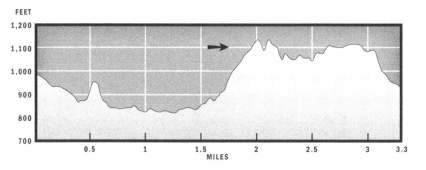

Rise into oak-dominated woods, huffing and puffing your way to reach a high point at 1.8 miles. Congratulations, you just climbed nearly 300 feet. Join the upper end of the bluff, heading westerly. The Clinch looks much smaller from up here! Watch for some sizeable oaks and creamy white dogwood blossoms in spring. Wintertime views open on the dam and Norris Lake to the north.

At 2.3 miles, come near a closed forest road in a gap. Continue your wooded forest walk. At 2.7 miles, the slender River Bluff Trail switchbacks sharply downhill. A second switchback hastens the descent, and at 3 miles you find yourself completing the loop portion of the hike. Backtrack 0.3 miles to the trailhead.

Nearby Attractions

Norris Dam and Norris Dam State Park are a stone's throw from this trail. Paddlers and anglers will be interested in plying the Clinch River, with its nationally recognized tailwater trout fishery. The chilly Clinch makes a fun float for non-anglers as well, when Norris Dam is generating.

Directions

From Exit 128 (Lake City) on I-75 north of Knoxville, take US 441 south 3.8 miles, then turn right on Dabney Lane, before Norris Dam but after Norris Dam State Park. Follow Dabney Lane just a few feet, then veer left on a paved road heading downhill, with a sign indicating Norris Dam. Follow the paved road 0.7 miles to end at a gate and the River Bluff Trail trailhead.

THE CUMBERLAND PLATEAU CAN BE A ROCKY PLACE.

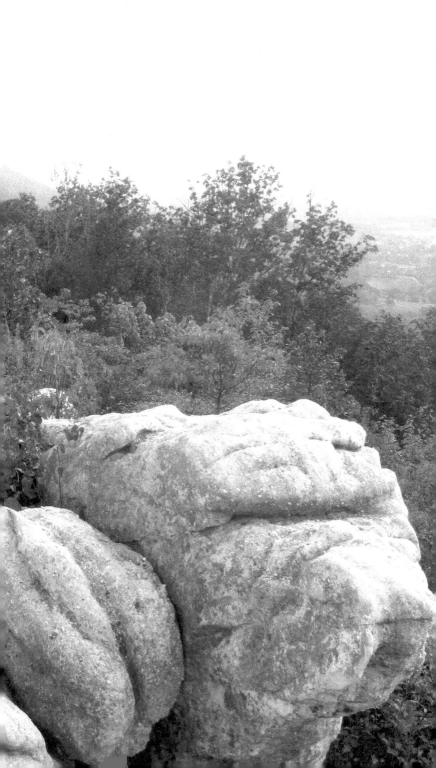

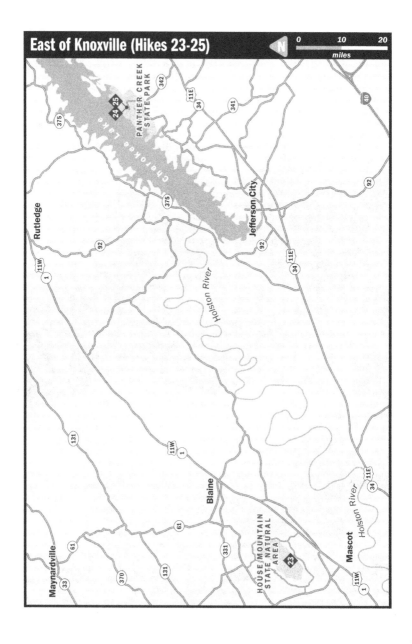

East

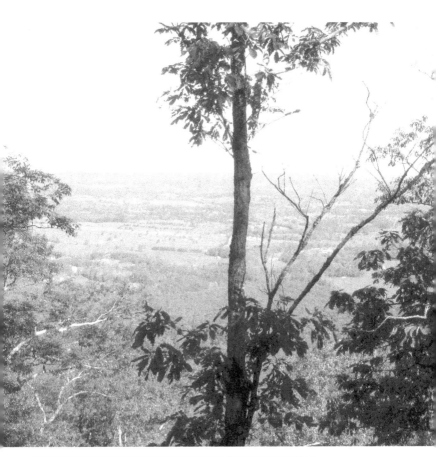

SPECTACULAR VIEWS AWAIT ON MANY HIKES EAST OF KNOXVILLE.

SCENERY: ★ ★ ★ ★
TRAIL CONDITION: ★ ★
CHILDREN: ★ ★
DIFFICULTY: ★ ★ ★
SOLITUDE: ★ ★

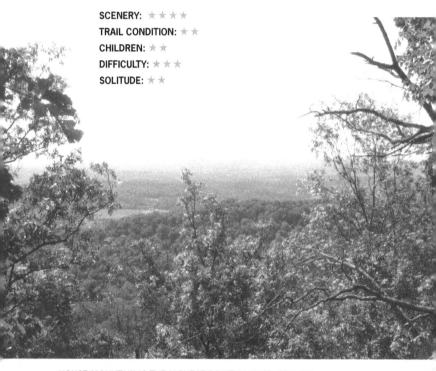

HOUSE MOUNTAIN IS THE HIGHEST POINT IN KNOX COUNTY.

GPS TRAILHEAD COORDINATES: N36° 6.286' W83° 45.775'

DISTANCE & CONFIGURATION: 2.9-mile loop

HIKING TIME: 1.8 hours

HIGHLIGHTS: Mountain vistas, birding area

ELEVATION: 1,200 feet at trailhead to 1,950 feet at West Overlook

ACCESS: No fees, permits, or passes required; open dawn to dusk

MAPS: House Mountain State Natural Area, USGS John Sevier

FACILITIES: Restrooms, shaded picnic shelter

WHEELCHAIR ACCESS: None

COMMENTS: Other short trails lie at the base of House Mountain.

CONTACTS: Knoxville Parks and Recreation, 2447 Sutherland Ave., Knoxville, TN 37919; (865) 215-6600; **ci.knoxville.tn.us/parks**

Overview

This loop takes you to a pair of vistas atop the highest point in Knox County—House Mountain. House Mountain stands in a 500-acre state natural area and is a steep-sloped, very rocky outlier peak. The geology reveals sheer bluffs, big boulders, rock houses, and, of course, stony overlooks where you can see in all four cardinal directions from various points on the mountain. The views attract hikers but also birders. Be apprised the hike is steep in areas and part of the mountain contains private property.

Route Details

House Mountain is a great addition to the hiking opportunities in greater Knoxville. Area mountain hiking usually takes place on the Cumberland Plateau or in the Smoky Mountains. House Mountain, a lone physiographic entity, used to be part of Clinch Mountain (which you can see from the East Overlook), but over time Big Flat Creek wore away the land, leaving House Mountain to itself. Now, not only can you see the landmarks of East Tennessee from House Mountain—such as the Smokies, downtown Knoxville, and the Cumberlands—but House Mountain is a landmark itself. And yes, it does have a house shape, which can be seen very distinctly on I-40 heading east from Knoxville.

The state-owned parcel is managed by Knox County. A restroom and shaded picnic pavilion enhance the trailhead. A reminder: the climb from the trailhead to the crest of House Mountain is short but steep. Be mentally prepared. Depart from the trailhead on the Connector Trail, and Left Sawmill Loop soon leaves left. Immediately pass under a power line and reenter hardwoods of red maple, white oak, redbud, and hickory. Reach a trail junction at 0.1 mile. Stay left, joining West Overlook Trail. You will climb 700 feet in a 0.8-mile distance. The rocky singletrack path makes its way uphill along Hogskin Branch, which drains the southern reaches of House Mountain. By the way, as this side of House Mountain faces south,

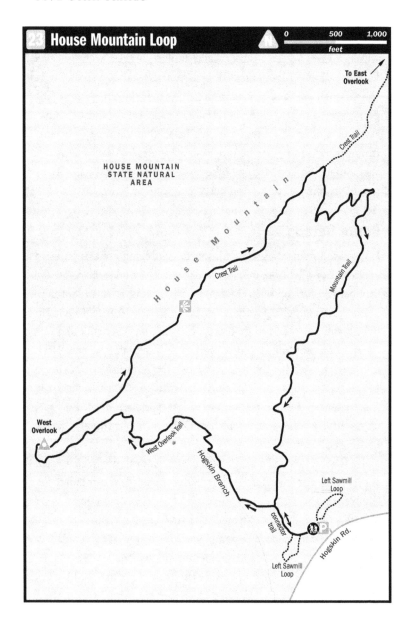

it can be brutally hot on a summer afternoon. If visiting during the warm season, try to start your hike in the morning. Also, brush may crowd the narrow path in the growing season. The climb is moderated by numerous switchbacks; it is the actual slope of the mountain that is so steep. Parts of this trail system have suffered terrible erosion, so please do not shortcut the switchbacks; fences help prevent hikers from doing so. The extreme slope of the mountain is such that erosive runoff is extra damaging.

By 0.5 miles, you have left Hogskin Branch, angling westerly for the west side of House Mountain. By 0.7 miles you are just below the mountain crest in extremely rocky woods of pine, oak, and sassafras, with an irregular stony cliff line standing above. Come alongside a pair of rock houses at 0.8 miles. The first is small. Watch for small, gnarled hickory trees clinging to the thin soils between boulders. Views open between the trees to the south. At 0.9 miles the trail curves around the west point of the mountain, angling uphill between boulders to emerge at the West Overlook. Explore a series of multilevel rock protrusions offering vistas primarily to the west, where downtown Knoxville rises.

Beyond the West Overlook the loop travels easterly, now on the Crest Trail, through lichen-covered boulders amid cedar, pine, and hickory woods. Obscured views of the Cumberland Plateau open north through the pines. The steep climb is over, and the Crest Trail

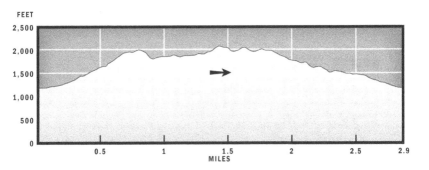

143

undulates past a pair of repose benches at 1.1 miles. The path then picks up an old roadbed and becomes wide and easy as it follows the contours of House Mountain. At 1.3 miles, a short spur trail leads left to a stellar view. Here, hikers are rewarded with clear views of the rolling hills below, Norris Lake in the distance, and Cumberland Mountain rising beyond that. Reach an old roadbed just beyond the overlook and stay left, wandering under a transmission line. Keep northeasterly, passing a couple of old roads leading left; one is to private property.

The path descends on a sand, clay, and dirt path to reach a trail junction at 1.7 miles. Here, the Crest Trail keeps northeasterly 0.7 miles to the East Overlook, where you can see Clinch Mountain and beyond. However, if you continue to the East Overlook, the trail runs near private property and you may see ATV riders. Please don't harass them and respect private property rights. This loop turns right and descends on the Mountain Trail. The slope shortly becomes insanely steep, and the singletrack trail does the best it can to mitigate the slope with switchbacks that navigate wooded rock bluffs. Views open to the south of the Smoky Mountains. The going is slow, so just take your time and enjoy the views. At 2.1 miles, pass a closed mountain access trail coming from the lowlands. At 2.3 miles, the trail briefly turns uphill, then bisects the first of several wet-weather streambeds. Watch for big boulders in the woods before completing the loop portion of the hike at 2.8 miles. Backtrack 0.1 mile to the trailhead.

Nearby Attractions

Two short lowland trails emanate from the trailhead: Left Sawmill Loop and Right Sawmill Loop. Each is about 0.25 miles long and both travel flats below the mountain, which presents wildflowers in early spring.

Directions

From Exit 392 on I-40 east of downtown Knoxville, take US 11W north 10.2 miles to Idumea Road. Turn left on Idumea and follow it 0.6 miles to Hogskin Road. Turn left on Hogskin Road and follow it 0.7 miles to the trailhead on your right.

24

Panther Creek State Park: Maple Arch Double Loop

SCENERY: ★ ★ ★ ★ ★
TRAIL CONDITION: ★ ★ ★ ★
CHILDREN: ★ ★
DIFFICULTY: ★ ★
SOLITUDE: ★ ★ ★

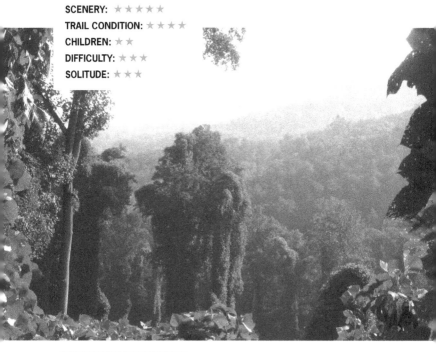

KUDZU-COVERED MOUNTAINS

GPS TRAILHEAD COORDINATES: N36° 12.971' W83° 24.338'

DISTANCE & CONFIGURATION: 5.5-mile double loop

HIKING TIME: 2.6 hours

HIGHLIGHTS: Mine vestiges, lake views

ELEVATION: 1,120 feet at trailhead to 1,410 feet at high point

ACCESS: No fees, permits, or passes required; open 8 a.m.–sunset

MAPS: Panther Creek State Park, USGS Talbott

FACILITIES: Restrooms, picnic shelter, picnic area

WHEELCHAIR ACCESS: None

COMMENTS: The state park campground is within walking distance of the trailhead.

CONTACTS: Panther Creek State Park, 2010 Panther Creek Rd., Morristown, TN 37814; (423) 587-7046; **tnstateparks.com**

Overview

Make two loops while exploring the hills of Panther Creek State Park, located on the shore of big Cherokee Lake. Follow the Ore Mine Trail up to River Ridge, then drop to the lake's edge. Here, you will trace the shoreline before ascending back into hills. A final stretch takes you past several sinkholes located amidst big wooded boulder fields.

Route Details

This view-filled hike has many ups and downs, never too long as to be exhausting yet long enough to get your lungs working. During its two-loop trek the hike passes through numerous environments: lakeshore, boulder fields, cedar thickets, pine woods, cove hardwoods, and even a kudzu stand. Avoid this trail on summer weekends, as that is when motorboats and personal watercraft will be tooling noisily all over the place. In winter you will have solitude and also may see waterfowl.

The Panther Creek State Park trail system is well signed and maintained. The parking area offers restrooms, a covered picnic shelter, and shaded picnic tables. The hike begins with an uphill grade. Pick up Ore Mine Trail at the upper end of the parking area. Lost Road Trail leads right. Pines and cedars rise from the rocky woods. Paw paws cluster in a draw on trail left. An impressive boulder field rises to your right. Step over the draw to make a trail junction at 0.2 miles. Stay right with the Ore Mine Trail, continuing up the hollow. It is here you will see shallow pits and gullies from a small-scale early 1800s manganese mining operation. Imagine how primitive the extraction techniques were compared to mines of today. Trees, vines, and vegetation cover the area, which has recovered well.

Make a sharp switchback at 0.5 miles, trying to surmount River Ridge. The singletrack hiker-only path tops out on River Ridge at a covered bench and four-way trail junction at 0.7 miles. Take Lost Road Trail, heading north on a downgrade through maples. It soon turns west toward Cherokee Lake, wandering into boulder-littered hickory, oak, and cedar woods. Avoid the shortcuts other hikers are

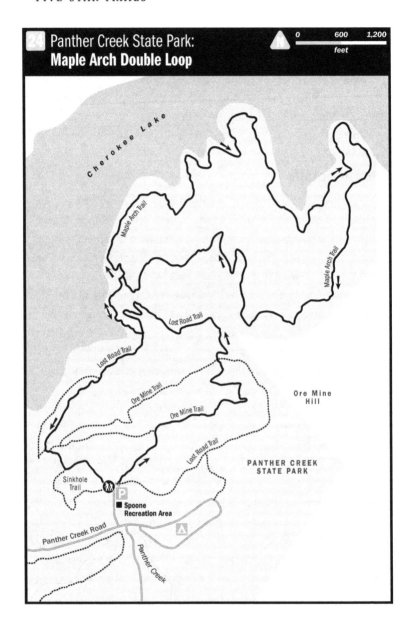

24 Panther Creek State Park:
Maple Arch Double Loop

0   600   1,200
feet

making as you switchback down the hill. Reach a signed trail junction at 1.2 miles. Turn right here, joining Maple Arch Trail. Cherokee Lake is now within rock-throwing distance. The lake is a large TVA impoundment, dammed near Jefferson City, that stretches clear up to Rogersville. The Holston River and its tributaries feed Cherokee. Below the lake dam, the Holston continues into Knoxville, where it meets the French Broad to form the Tennessee River.

Begin an extended stretch of lakeshore walking. Ahead, at 1.3 miles, spur trails lead left to the water. When the lake is below full pool, a gravel beach is exposed here, luring trail users to the lake. At 1.5 miles you will reach the actual loop portion of the Maple Arch Trail. Stay left here, continuing along the shoreline, enjoying lake views and also vistas of the many islands that rise from the impoundment. Curve around a drainage at 1.8 miles. Cedars and scrub pines pock the thin, stony soil. The trail goes off and on old roads abandoned after the Holston River was dammed to create Cherokee Lake.

Lake views persist, and Clinch Mountain forms a backdrop to Cherokee. At 2.4 miles, rise from the shoreline as you circle around an embayment. Step over the streambed that creates the embayment at 2.7 miles. Just below the trail, look for the stone remnants of an old primitive bridge crossing the wet-weather stream. Circle around a nearly level peninsula and recovering farm field and homesite. Leave

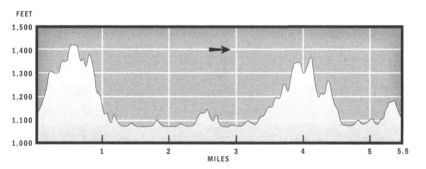

the lakeshore near the park boundary at 3.2 miles. The trail climbs into rocky woods, then passes through a boulder field before entering a moist hollow where the scenery changes yet again to cove hardwoods, such as tulip trees. Vines grow in tangles among the trees. For good measure, the path passes by an invasive kudzu stand at 4 miles.

Climb by switchbacks away from the weeds over a ridge, then drift westerly to complete the loop portion of the Maple Arch Trail at 4.6 miles. Be prepared for numerous junctions while working your way back to Spoone Recreation Area. Backtrack 0.2 miles along the lakeshore to rejoin the Lost Road Trail as it scales a hillside well above the water. The trail splits at 5 miles. Stay left with the hiker-only portion of the path through boulders.

Reach a four-way junction at 5.3 miles. Keep straight, still on Lost Road Trail, toward the parking area. You are in an incredible boulder field, surrounded by maple, redbud, hickory, and cedars galore. Reach the Sinkhole Trail at 5.4 miles. You can go right or left on this short loop. A left leads downhill through boulders to a big sink on trail left, at the base of the boulder field. Emerge at the Spoone Recreation Area near the restrooms at 5.5 miles.

Nearby Attractions

The state park has plentiful trails for hikers, bikers, and equestrians; boating; and a campground adjacent to this hike.

Directions

From Knoxville, take US 11E north to Morristown and the intersection of 11E and Panther Creek Road/TN 342. Turn left on TN 342 west. Follow it 2.4 miles, then turn right into the state park. Keep straight, passing the visitor center. At 0.7 miles, just past the right turn into the campground, turn right into a large parking area at the Spoone shelter. The hike starts at the upper end of the parking area in the auto turnaround.

25

Panther Creek State Park: Point Lookout Loop

SCENERY: ★ ★ ★ ★ ★
TRAIL CONDITION: ★ ★ ★
CHILDREN: ★ ★
DIFFICULTY: ★ ★ ★
SOLITUDE: ★ ★

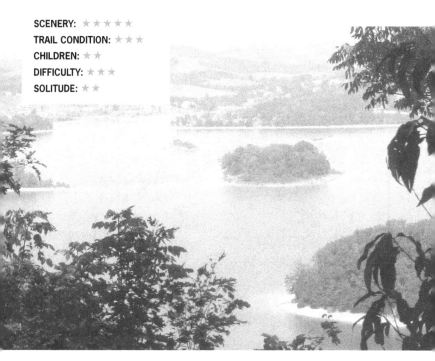

CHEROKEE LAKE

GPS TRAILHEAD COORDINATES: N36° 12.633' W83° 25.387'

DISTANCE & CONFIGURATION: 5.1-mile loop

HIKING TIME: 2.5 hours

HIGHLIGHTS: Multiple lake views from shoreline and hilltops

ELEVATION: 1,290 feet at trailhead to 1,470 feet at high point

ACCESS: No fees, permits, or passes; open 8 a.m.–sunset

MAPS: Panther Creek State Park, USGS Talbott

FACILITIES: Restrooms, picnic shelter, picnic area

WHEELCHAIR ACCESS: None

COMMENTS: The state park has miles of additional trails.

CONTACTS: Panther Creek State Park, 2010 Panther Creek Rd., Morristown, TN 37814; (423) 587-7046; **tnstateparks.com**

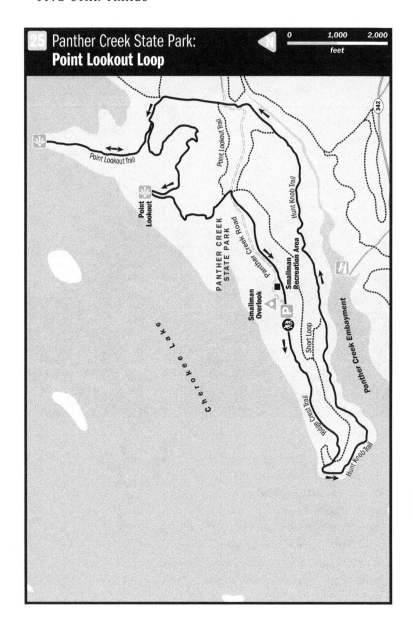

Overview

This view-laden trek starts with a trip through an amazing boulder garden on a slender but steep peninsula before dropping to Cherokee Lake. Drink in the watery vista before turning up Panther Creek embayment. Make a side trip to another shoreline with a view. Next, climb a high knob to absorb a first-rate panorama from aptly named Point Lookout. A final short road walk through an elongated picnic area takes you back to your vehicle.

Route Details

You will be happily surprised with this hike. It starts atop a scenic peninsula with an alluring picnic area. Bring a meal for before or after your hike. Walk a rocky spine with drop-offs on both sides, dipping to Cherokee Lake. Cruise along the narrowing embayment of the park's namesake, Panther Creek, before heading to another part of the lake. Make a side trip to a secluded peninsula. The final part of the trek winds up to Point Lookout, where you peer over the lake and beyond to mountains from a precipitous drop-off. Wander a short piece back to the trailhead.

Pick up Ridge Crest Trail at the western dead-end turnaround of Smallman Recreation Area. You will have to walk a bit from the parking area to reach the actual trail beginning. Enter a wooded

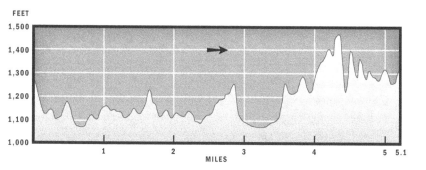

boulder garden, where pale rocks rise from a spare, gnarled forest of cedar, oak, and hickory. Watch for cacti growing in the thin, fast-draining soils. Surmount a knob, then resume a downgrade, meeting the Hunt Knob Trail. Keep straight to the lake and point of the peninsula, reaching a waterside vista at 0.7 miles. A gravel and rock drop-off allows you to access the lake, whether it is at full summer pool or lower winter levels. Stay left on the slender track, keeping the lake to your right, enjoying more aquatic views from the slope of a hill. Turn easterly into the ever-narrowing Panther Creek embayment. At 1.4 miles, the so-called Short Loop leaves left and circles back toward Ridge Crest Trail.

Pass a big sinkhole on trail left at 1.5 miles. Traverse some rugged boulder fields between shallow drainages. At 1.7 miles, just before a drainage, look on trail right for a rock cavity worn through at the bottom. Technically, this is an arch, but it may only be recognized as such by geologists. Look for willow trees growing in the upper Panther Creek embayment. Ahead, the slope eases. At 2.1 miles, the loop portion of Hunt Knob Trail leaves to the left. Keep straight, passing within earshot of flowing Panther Creek before turning into a grassy meadow and a trail junction at 2.3 miles. Stay left here, crossing the park road you drove in on.

Soon you'll reach yet another trail intersection. Here, Point Lookout Trail begins its loop, heading left and straight. Keep straight, tracing a wide gravel track on a gentle uptick in shady woods. Top out in a gap and trail junction at 2.5 miles. Stay left on Point Lookout Trail, gaining ground to reach a split at 2.7 miles. Here, enjoy your choice of views. Turn right, aiming for an isolated peninsula jutting north into Cherokee Lake. This half-mile spur ends at a point where you can gaze toward islands and beyond to the far lakeshore. This makes a great picnic spot if you want to lunch on the trail. A gravel beach grown up with persimmon trees is exposed at low winter lake levels. Remember this view to contrast it with your next vista, 400 feet higher. Backtrack uphill to the Point Lookout Loop, resuming a climb and breaking through a boulder field at 4 miles. Continue the uptick in maples, reaching Point Lookout at 4.3 miles. Here, a covered bench offers a seat. Soak in panoramas opening to the northwest of the island-studded impoundment and Clinch Mountain beyond. The vista is easily worth the ascent.

Cruise southwesterly toward the trailhead, meandering downhill to reach a gap and trail junction at 4.7 miles. Here, the other end of Point Lookout Trail comes in from your left. However, this hike keeps straight to shortly emerge on the park road that brought you in. Turn right here, walking west along a grassy roadside strip. The first picnic area loop is just ahead, while the second picnic area loop, with Smallman Overlook, is reached at 5.1 miles, ending the hike.

Nearby Attractions

The state park has plentiful trails for hikers, bikers, and equestrians; boating; and a campground adjacent to this hike.

Directions

From Knoxville, take US 11E north to Morristown and the intersection of 11E and Panther Creek Road/TN 342. Turn left on TN 342 west. Follow it 2.4 miles, then turn right into the state park. Keep straight, passing the visitor center. Continue past the campground to reach Smallman Recreation Area after 1.8 miles. Continue past Smallman Overlook to park. No parking is allowed in the auto turnaround at the actual trailhead.

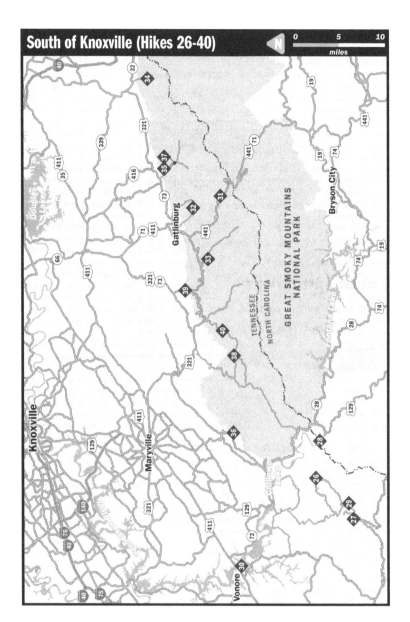

South

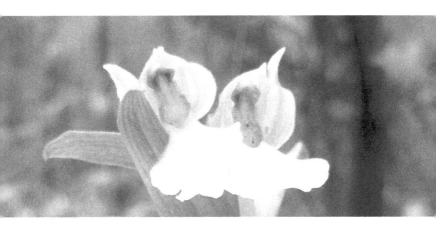

SHOWY ORCHIS

26

Cherokee National Forest:
Crowder Place via Fodderstack

SCENERY: ★ ★ ★
TRAIL CONDITION: ★ ★ ★
CHILDREN: ★ ★
DIFFICULTY: ★ ★ ★
SOLITUDE: ★ ★ ★ ★

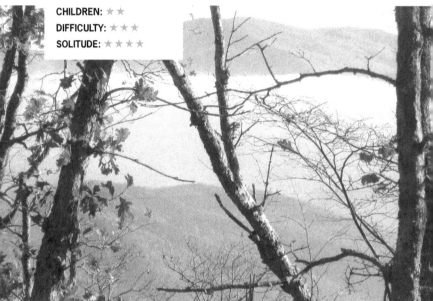

LOOKING OUT FROM FODDERSTACK RIDGE

GPS TRAILHEAD COORDINATES: N35° 27.800' W84° 1.643'

DISTANCE & CONFIGURATION: 6.8-mile out-and-back

HIKING TIME: 3.5 hours

HIGHLIGHTS: Views of Smokies, old homesite

ELEVATION: 2,830 feet at trailhead to 3,650 feet at high point

ACCESS: No fees, permits, or passes required

MAPS: Cherokee National Forest–Tellico & Ocoee Rivers; USGS Whiteoak Flats

FACILITIES: None

WHEELCHAIR ACCESS: None

CONTACTS: Cherokee National Forest, 2800 North Ocoee St., Cleveland, TN 37312; (423) 476-9700; **fs.fed.us/r8/cherokee**

Overview

Make a ridgetop run in the Citico Wilderness, just south of the Smokies in Monroe County. Head south in rich woods along Fodderstack Mountain, where views open on Gregory Bald and the western Smoky Mountains. Follow the undulating ridge to a gap, where you drop to a flat and spring, marking the homesite known as Crowder Place. Grab some fresh spring water and relax before backtracking to the trailhead.

Route Details

You get to enjoy not one but two federally designated wildernesses on this hike. The ridge you will be following, Fodderstack Mountain, marks the boundary between Citico Creek Wilderness, which is entirely in Tennessee, and Joyce Kilmer Slickrock Wilderness, which is mostly in North Carolina. Practically speaking, this means your views from the ridgetop will be of natural mountain lands cloaked in rich woods. This would be a great destination on fall weekends when the Smokies roads and trails are extremely busy.

Leave Farr Gap and walk just a few feet to reach a trail intersection and kiosk. Here, Stiffknee Trail leaves left and downhill toward Slickrock Creek. The Fodderstack Trail stays right and uphill under maples and tulip trees. Curve around a point at 0.3 miles. You are gaining the top of the ridge to make a southeasterly course in drier woods of hickory, chestnut, oak, pines, and blueberries. Top out at 0.6 miles and begin undulating along the crest. Views open between the trees to the north, and you can make out the peaks of the Smokies. Look for the field of Gregory Bald, which will be visible on clear fall and winter days. Views also open toward the west of the greater Tennessee Valley. The distinct sharp face of Hangover Lead to the southeast rises across Slickrock Creek Valley. Note the signs indicating this area is a bear reserve.

Reach a gap at 1 mile. Begin an extended uptick toward Little Fodderstack. Curve around the west side of the peak, never quite

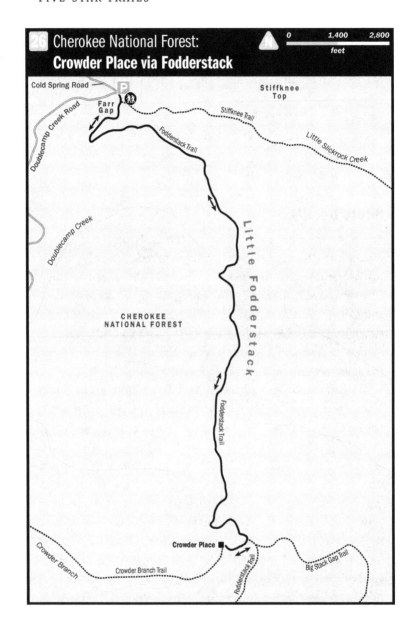

reaching the top, but instead bypassing the high point in striped maples, then coming to a gap. Regain the now narrow ridge crest at 2 miles. To your left is the watershed of Slickrock Creek, and to your right is the watershed of Citico Creek. Continue rolling along the ridge, passing through another gap at 2.5 miles. Trek over a final knob. The now-sandy trail makes a half-loop, moderating its descent to reach another gap and trail junction at 3.3 miles. Here, Trail #84, Crowder Branch Trail, leaves right and descends, while Fodderstack Trail keeps straight. Big Stack Gap Trail leaves left a short piece down Fodderstack Trail. Take Crowder Branch Trail downhill into the remnants of a surprisingly persistent field. Look for a couple of scrubby old apple trees as you pass what once was a farm field maintained by the Crowder family, then by the U.S. Forest Service as a wildlife clearing until the Citico Creek Wilderness was established in 1984. I have been coming here for more than two decades, and the field gets a little smaller and the trees a little bigger every visit. In summer, the brush may nearly obscure the trail as it passes through what's left of the field.

Reach Crowder Place at 3.4 miles. It is located in a flat between two branches. Look for rock frame outlines of their homestead in the grassy area. You can also see the developed spring if you walk up the right-hand draw. Backpackers use Crowder Place as a campsite, and there is usually a fire ring set up. Of course the Crowders had a

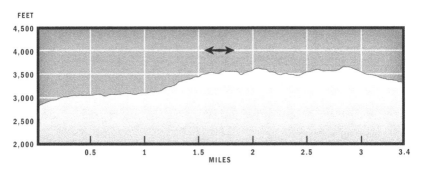

fireplace for cooking and heating their wooden cabin. Winters were cold and long here at 3,300 feet in these Tennessee mountains. Rest and relax, allowing time to absorb the atmosphere and imagine what it was like living up here day after day, year after year, a century ago. Look around for old metal artifacts but leave them for others to discover and enjoy. Note the Crowder Branch Trail continues downstream to reach Doublecamp Road. (You could walk down it 2.4 miles, then follow Forest Road 2659 for 2.5 miles up to Farr Gap, creating an 8.3-mile loop.)

Nearby Attractions

Citico Wilderness and Joyce Kilmer Slickrock Wilderness offer miles and miles of primitive trails with elevations ranging from 1,100 feet to more than 5,000 feet.

Directions

From Knoxville, take US 129/Alcoa Highway south through Maryville and join US 411 south of Maryville, heading toward Madisonville. Bridge the impounded Tellico River, coming to Vonore. Look for the intersection with TN 360 at a traffic light. Turn left on TN 360 south and drive 12.9 miles to Monroe County 504/Chestnut Valley Road (also known as Buck Highway). A sign to Citico Creek will mark your left turn. After the left turn, drive 5.1 miles to FS 35-1/Citico Creek Road. Along the way, make sure to veer left at the intersection with Monroe County 506. After turning right on FS 35-1, drive 6.4 miles to reach Doublecamp camping area and Forest Road 2659, just before a bridge. Turn left and join FR 2659/Doublecamp Road and follow it 6.3 miles to end at Farr Gap. The Fodderstack Trail starts on the right as you reach the gap. Parking is on the right-hand side just below Farr Gap.

27

Cherokee National Forest:
Indian Boundary Lake Loop

SCENERY: ★ ★ ★ ★
TRAIL CONDITION: ★ ★ ★ ★ ★
CHILDREN: ★ ★ ★ ★
DIFFICULTY: ★
SOLITUDE: ★ ★

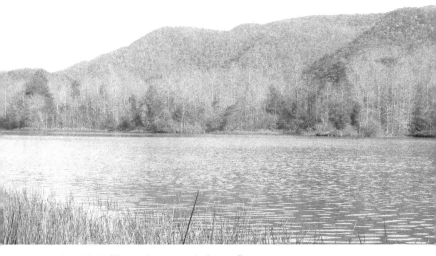

MOUNTAINS RISE FROM INDIAN BOUNDARY LAKE.

GPS TRAILHEAD COORDINATES: N35° 23.915' W84° 6.657'

DISTANCE & CONFIGURATION: 3.1-mile loop

HIKING TIME: 1.5 hours

HIGHLIGHTS: Lake and mountain views in outstanding recreation area

ELEVATION: 1,780 feet at trailhead to 1,800 feet at high point

ACCESS: No fees, permits, or passes required; campground open April–October

MAPS: Cherokee National Forest–Tellico & Ocoee Rivers, USGS Whiteoak Flats

FACILITIES: Restrooms and water at picnic area and campground

WHEELCHAIR ACCESS: Yes, all-access trail

CONTACTS: Cherokee National Forest, 2800 North Ocoee St., Cleveland, TN 37312; (423) 476-9700; **fs.fed.us/r8/cherokee**

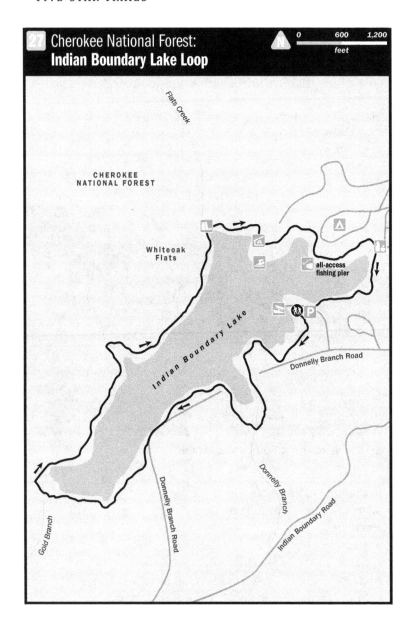

Overview

Make a loop at this scenic Cherokee National Forest impoundment. Located in Whiteoak Flats below Flats Mountain, explore Indian Boundary Recreation Area via this all-access, nearly level loop trail. Leave the boat ramp and walk past man-made fishing peninsulas, bridging numerous streams shaded in rhododendron. Views open on the lake but also on Flats Mountain, which rises on one side of Indian Boundary. Great camping, swimming, and fishing can also be enjoyed at this mountain retreat.

Route Details

Indian Boundary is the pride of the Cherokee National Forest. And with good reason—the area lies in a flat beside a clear lake and beneath tall mountains. Hikers can enjoy the recreation area on this pleasant and easy loop doable by nearly everyone. A coat of pea gravel covers the trail bed. The scant undulations are graded for wheelchairs. So even when you and the family have polished off a buffet after church, the whole clan could still take on this trail. And from a visual standpoint you get to enjoy mountain views and scenery without the ruggedness that so often accompanies mountain treks.

Leave the boat ramp, traveling southwesterly with Indian Boundary Lake to your right. A xeric forest of hickory, pine, sweetgum,

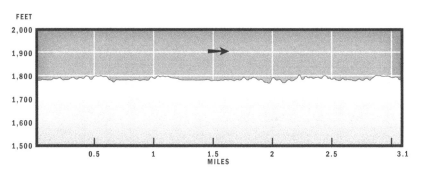

and oak shades the level path as it travels through the area known as Whiteoak Flats. And flat it is. Bridge a pair of streamlets at 0.1 mile, then pass through a meadow. Return to the lakeside. You can already look back at the boat ramp and across the lake at the swim beach. Watery views are nearly continuous, albeit sometimes through the trees. Pass the first of several soil fishing peninsulas that extend to the water. Note the non-native cypress trees planted on these peninsulas.

Bridge Donnelly Branch at 0.5 miles after working around its embayment. Bisect another grassy meadow. These are wildlife clearings maintained by the forest service. These clearings create "edges," where different ecotones overlap, allowing more food for animals. For example, blackberries grow on the edges of such clearings. Pass an angler's access road at 0.9 miles. At 1 mile, come near gated Donnelly Branch Road, but stay with the pea gravel track and you'll be fine.

Begin circling around the upper lake, bridging Gold Branch and Flats Creek. Watch for evidence of beaver dams here. Turn back northeasterly. Views open of Flats Mountain, which majestically rises from the far shoreline. Big white pines shade the path. You are close to the shore and may see paddlers in canoes and kayak as well as fishermen in johnboats. Circle around an embayment and tributary at 1.8 miles.

At 2.1 miles you are directly across from the boat ramp where you started. Bridge the lake dam at 2.2 miles. Come to the swim beach pavilion, with water and restrooms, at 2.4 miles. Begin cruising by the campground, passing coveted lakeside sites. Watch out for social trails leading to camps. Reach the metal all-access fishing pier at 2.6 miles. If you are thirsty, stop at the camp store (open in season) at 2.8 miles. You are in the home stretch. Reach the boat ramp access road at 3.1 miles, completing the hike.

After seeing Indian Boundary you may want to camp here. Individual campsites are tastefully integrated into the natural beauty of the land. Amenities include warm showers, electricity at some sites, and flush toilets. Anglers enjoy bank fishing or launching a boat into the clear waters for largemouth bass, trout, and bream. There are purportedly some tackle-busting catfish down deep. You passed the alluring swim beach. Your entrance road, the Cherohala Skyway, rivals the Blue Ridge Parkway or Newfound Gap Road in the Smokies for scenery. Panoramic overlooks dot the way to Beech Gap and beyond the North Carolina state line. Stop at Hooper Bald. Take a short nature trail to reach this meadow at 5,300 feet in elevation. Indian Boundary is a popular camping destination. If you want to camp, consider making reservations or coming in May, when spring runs rampant. Fall is also a good choice; the Cherohala Skyway traverses elevations low and high, so leaf viewers are likely to see vibrant colors.

Nearby Attractions

Nearby Citico Wilderness offers miles and miles of primitive trails with elevations ranging from 1,100 feet to more than 5,000 feet.

Directions

From Knoxville, take US 129/Alcoa Highway south through Maryville and join US 411 south of Maryville, heading to Madisonville. Join TN 68 south to Tellico Plains. From Tellico Plains, pick up TN 165/Cherohala Skyway and drive 14 miles to Forest Road 345. Turn left on FR 345 and follow it 1.2 miles into the Indian Boundary Recreation Area. Enter the recreation area, then turn left at a split toward the boat ramp. Turn into the boat ramp area and park there. The trail leaves left from the boat ramp as you face Indian Boundary Lake.

28

Cherokee National
Forest: Slickrock Creek Loop

SCENERY:	★ ★ ★ ★
TRAIL CONDITION:	★ ★ ★
CHILDREN:	★ ★
DIFFICULTY:	★ ★ ★
SOLITUDE:	★ ★

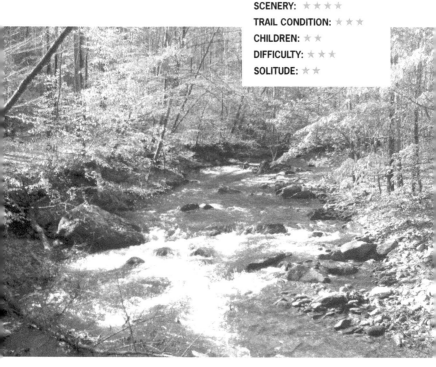

SLICKROCK CREEK

GPS TRAILHEAD COORDINATES: N35° 26.953' W83° 56.517'

DISTANCE & CONFIGURATION: 6.4-mile balloon loop

HIKING TIME: 4 hours

HIGHLIGHTS: Lower Falls, Slickrock Creek

ELEVATION: 1,140 feet at trailhead to 1,840 feet at high point

ACCESS: No fees, permits, or passes required

MAPS: Cherokee National Forest–Tellico & Ocoee Rivers, USGS Tapoco

FACILITIES: None

WHEELCHAIR ACCESS: None

CONTACTS: Cherokee National Forest, 2800 North Ocoee St., Cleveland, TN 37312; (423) 476-9700; **fs.fed.us/r8/cherokee**

Overview

Make a wilderness loop along raucous Slickrock Creek, a wild mountain watercourse framed in wooded beauty. You will first walk above serpentine Calderwood Lake, then turn into the Smokies-esque stream. The first of two fords leads to Lower Falls; with its huge pool, it's a draw for summertime swimmers. Finally, climb away from the stream and make a circuit back to Calderwood Lake, where a short backtrack returns you to the trailhead.

Route Details

This is a great alternative to the Smokies. The scenery is more similar than not. On your drive in you will wind your way through US 129, "The Dragon" of motorcycling fame. You will also pass Cheoah Dam, where scenes from the movie *The Fugitive* were filmed. Once at the trailhead, enter Joyce Kilmer Slickrock Wilderness, a federally designated wildland encompassing parts of Tennessee's Cherokee National Forest and North Carolina's Nantahala National Forest. For the entire time you are following Slickrock Creek it actually forms the boundary between the Volunteer State and the Tar Heel State.

Pick up a doubletrack path, Slickrock Creek Trail, with Calderwood Lake to your right. The clear, clean impoundment of the Little Tennessee River makes a silent, snake-like course below. A steep wooded hillside rises to your left. Dense hardwoods of birch, beech, tulip trees, and maples grow where they can in the rocky soil. At 0.5 miles the trail devolves from doubletrack to singletrack. At 0.6 miles, Ike Branch Trail leaves left. This is your return route.

Keep straight on Slickrock Creek Trail, stepping over Ike Branch. Join an even steeper slope as the path works around rock promontories and bluffs. Occasional wooden bridges help you negotiate the steepest of bluffs. Curve into Slickrock Creek embayment. Views open to the north of the lake. The watery intimations of Slickrock Creek drift to your ears. Drop to reach the stream at 1.8 miles. You will turn up the creek on a primitive wilderness-grade trail. Even as

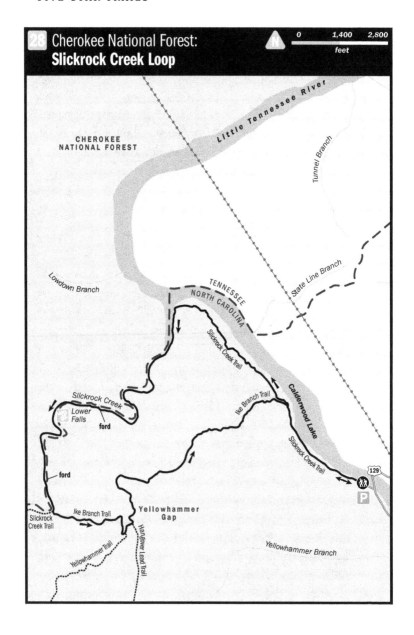

28 Cherokee National Forest:
Slickrock Creek Loop

N

0   1,400   2,800
feet

CHEROKEE
NATIONAL FOREST

Little Tennessee River

Tunnel Branch

Lowdown Branch

TENNESSEE
NORTH CAROLINA

State Line Branch

Slickrock Creek Trail

Slickrock Creek

Lower
Falls

ford

Ike Branch Trail

Calderwood Lake

Slickrock Creek Trail

ford

129

Slickrock
Creek Trail

Ike Branch Trail

Yellowhammer
Gap

P

Yellowhammer Trail

Hangover Lead Trail

Yellowhammer Branch

you navigate your way, the beauty of the creek cannot be denied: crystalline water flowing over boulders, rich vegetation growing on anything that doesn't move, mountain slopes rising to the sky, trout-filled pools, tree-covered islands, and waterside gravel bars. An overabundance of campsites is the only downside. Anglers might want to bring a fishing pole. As the creek is the state line, a Tennessee fishing license and trout stamp are valid.

Keep upstream as the trail passes alternately through bottomland and along bluffs that make passage challenging. The watercourse bends, and you trace those bends, going on and off an old railroad bed. At 2.7 miles, come to the first ford of Slickrock Creek. A stout stick helps here. Cross over to the Tennessee side of the watercourse, keeping upstream. At 2.9 miles, pass below at a tributary forming a small trailside waterfall. Reach Lower Falls at 3 miles. Here, Slickrock Creek pours over a wide stone lip about 15 feet into one of the larger pools in the Southern Appalachians. In summer you will be tempted to jump in and cool off. The large pool also allows ample sunlight to spill onto the stream. Large flat boulders provide sunning spots beside the falls.

Leave the roaring cataract behind, continuing upriver. The plethora of campsites sometimes makes the route confusing, as spur paths will lead to the camps. Join a south-facing piney bluff before dropping to meet the second ford at 3.5 miles. This ford is a little more

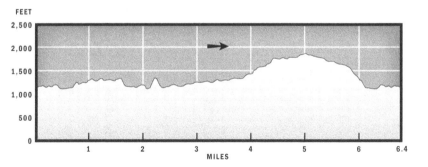

challenging, as it is deeper with an irregular stream bottom. Cross back over to North Carolina, continuing upstream among doghobble and rhododendron. Fight your way around a little gnarly bluff, then reach a campsite and trail junction at 3.7 miles. Look left as the somewhat-dim-yet-signed Ike Branch Trail leaves left away from Slickrock Creek and uphill. Step over a small branch and rise amid yellow birch, black birch, and buckeye. Keep hiking up the hollow to reach a trail intersection at 4.2 miles. Here, the Yellowhammer Trail leaves right. Stay left with the Ike Branch Trail, wandering the mountainside on a narrow path. The northbound path meets Hangover Lead Trail at 4.3 miles, just below Yellowhammer Gap. Continue straight on Ike Branch Trail beneath mid-slope dogwoods, oaks, and white pines. Pass through gaps at 4.6 miles and 5 miles. Dip into the intimate Ike Branch hollow. Cross Ike Branch a few times, then pass a homesite on your right. Piled rocks are all that remain of Ike's highland homestead. The path steepens before you open into the Little Tennessee River Valley. Come to Slickrock Creek Trail at 5.8 miles, completing the loop portion of the hike. Backtrack 0.6 miles to the trailhead.

Nearby Attractions

Joyce Kilmer Slickrock Wilderness offers miles and miles of primitive trails with elevations ranging from 1,100 feet to more than 5,000 feet.

Directions

From Knoxville, take US 129/Alcoa Highway south through Maryville and beyond to the North Carolina state line at Deals Gap. Stay with US 129 south to soon cross Calderwood Lake just below Cheoah Dam. Turn right into a parking area just after crossing Calderwood.

29

Cherokee National Forest:
South Fork Citico Sampler

SCENERY: ★ ★ ★ ★
TRAIL CONDITION: ★ ★ ★
CHILDREN: ★ ★ ★
DIFFICULTY: ★ ★
SOLITUDE: ★ ★ ★

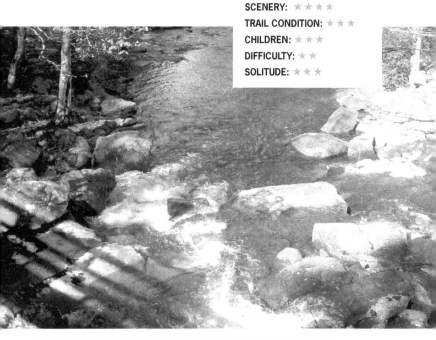

SOUTH FORK CITICO CREEK IS A QUINTESSENTIAL MOUNTAIN STREAM.

GPS TRAILHEAD COORDINATES: N35° 24.335' W84° 4.801'

DISTANCE & CONFIGURATION: 3.8-mile out-and-back

HIKING TIME: 2 hours

HIGHLIGHTS: Wilderness stream, swimming, fishing

ELEVATION: 1,720 feet at trailhead to 2,040 feet at turnaround point

ACCESS: No fees, permits, or passes required

MAPS: Cherokee National Forest–Tellico & Ocoee Rivers, USGS Whiteoak Flats

FACILITIES: Primitive campground near trailhead

WHEELCHAIR ACCESS: None

CONTACTS: Cherokee National Forest, 2800 North Ocoee St., Cleveland, TN 37312; (423) 476-9700; **fs.fed.us/r8/cherokee**

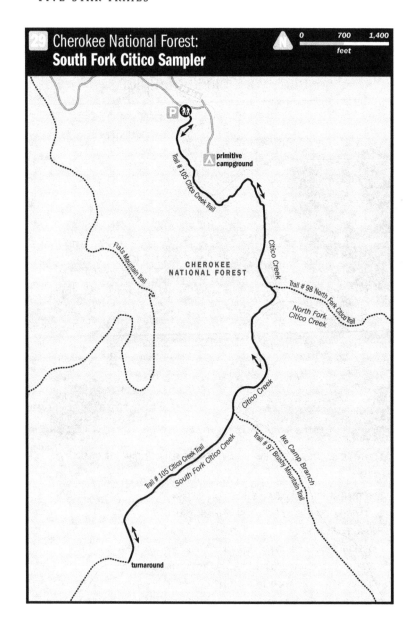

29 Cherokee National Forest:
South Fork Citico Sampler

0   700   1,400
feet

primitive
campground

Trail # 105 Citico Creek Trail

Flats Mountain Trail

CHEROKEE
NATIONAL FOREST

Citico Creek

Trail # 98 North Fork Citico Trail

North Fork
Citico Creek

Citico Creek

Trail # 105 Citico Creek Trail

South Fork Citico Creek

Trail # 97 Bushly Mountain Trail

Ike Camp Branch

turnaround

Overview

This hike explores the lowermost, gorgeous Citico Creek Wilderness, just south of the Smokies. Follow a foot trail past the confluence of North and South Fork Citico Creek. Continue up South Fork Citico Creek, with its continuous cascades, rapids, and shoals pouring over rocks and boulders into still and deep pools. The hike wanders up the valley for nearly 2 miles. As no stream fords are required for this part of the trail, you can enjoy it during all seasons—winter with its icy cascades, summer for swimming, spring for wildflowers, and fall for colors.

Route Details

This hike will tempt you to go beyond the mileage recommended in this book. It is that beautiful. South Fork Citico Creek is the centerpiece of the Citico Creek Wilderness. Located just south of Great Smoky Mountains National Park, the area offers scenery like the Smokies minus the crowds. However, the trails are a little rougher, and this lends a more primitive experience overall. That said, you will likely find the experience a good one and want to investigate not only this trail but other pathways in the 57-mile Citico Creek Wilderness trail system.

Pass around the vehicle barriers, joining Trail #105. Descend on a doubletrack into a flat. A primitive camping area lies across the

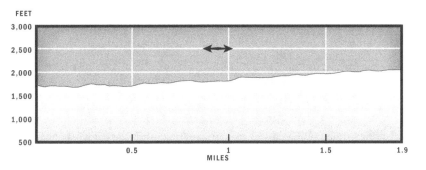

creek and is accessed by the concrete ford mentioned in the trailhead directions. Hikers often start at the primitive campground but end up having to ford Citico Creek to join the official trail.

After 0.25 miles, the path crosses a small rocky tributary. This path slims to a singletrack trail that soon becomes pinched by a steep bluff. Slip down to the water's edge. Look at the creek—rushing rapids fighting their way amidst mossy gray boulders, still eddies where water striders stand on the surface, fallen trees ceaselessly pushed by the current, bubbles from white froth oxygenating the water for wily trout. Vegetation grows to the shoreline, forming a natural green tunnel for Citico Creek. The sun penetrates where the stream is at its widest, and when the fallen leaves allow weak winter rays to shine through the translucent water—a classic Southern Appalachian mountain stream within a federally designated wilderness.

While hiking, watch for white quartz rocks brightening the woods. Open into a flat at 0.4 miles. This once brushy area is now growing up in trees. You may see structure foundations of what was purportedly an orchard. At 0.5 miles, a wooden sign welcomes you into the wilderness. A user-created trail comes in from the primitive campground across the creek. You are back along the stream. Sweetgum, red maple, Fraser magnolia, and sycamore shade the track. White pine, doghobble, and rhododendron add an evergreen touch to the biodiversity.

The ultra-clear water repeatedly lures you toward Citico Creek. At 0.7 miles, big open rock slabs beside some rapids provide the perfect opportunity to get close to the stream. Ahead, turn away from the creek. Even when you can't see the stream it is always within earshot. Join an old railroad grade. Unbelievably, this area was once connected to Maryville by rail. A logging operation built the system to extract timber from the Citico Creek watershed. Just ahead, you'll see a concrete building on your right. That is all that remains of the logging community of Jeffrey. Operations ceased in the 1920s when a huge fire burned up the infrastructure and woodlands. A few years later the area was purchased by the United States Forest Service, and over the decades it has healed into the land of spring wildflowers, summertime trout fishing, and fall kaleidoscope of color.

At 0.8 miles, come to a trail junction. Here, the North Fork Citico Trail, Trail #98, leaves left. Go ahead and take the trail and reach a bridge over Citico Creek. This offers an overhead vista of the mountain rill. The confluence of the North Fork and South Fork is within sight. Return to the South Fork Trail, Trail #105, and continue upstream, now tracing South Fork Citico Creek.

The tread has narrowed and you follow an old railroad bed. The unbroken beauty continues in pools and shoals. At 1.2 miles, you can see Ike Branch splashing its way to meet Citico Creek. At 1.3 miles, Brushy Mountain Trail, Trail #97, heads to the left but requires a ford of South Fork. Continue upstream. At 1.9 miles, the trail leads directly to an old ford of Citico Creek. This is a good place to turn around. However, a slender footpath leaves right, climbs a hill, and descends back to the creek, getting around two old fords and rejoining the old railroad grade after 0.5 miles before reaching the first mandatory ford of Citico Creek. On your return trip, find a good riverside rock and enjoy this watery jewel of East Tennessee.

Nearby Attractions

Nearby Citico Wilderness offers miles and miles of primitive trails with elevations ranging from 1,100 feet to more than 5,000 feet.

Directions

From Knoxville, take US 129/Alcoa Highway south through Maryville and join US 411 south of Maryville, heading toward Madisonville. Bridge the impounded Tellico River, coming to Vonore. Look for the intersection with TN 360 at a traffic light. Turn left on TN 360 south and drive 12.9 miles to Monroe County 504/Chestnut Valley Road (also known as Buck Highway). A sign to Citico Creek will mark your left turn. After the left turn, drive 5.1 miles to FS 35-1/Citico Creek Road. Turn right on FS 35-1, passing Doublecamp camping area at

6.4 miles. Keep straight here, crossing a bridge. At 8 miles, FS 35-1 makes a sharp right turn—a road splits left to a concrete ford over Citico Creek. Do not take that road; continue uphill 0.1 mile farther to the South Fork Citico Trail, Trail #105, trailhead. It is on your left, with a pair of big rock vehicle barriers. There is parking for one or two cars near the gate or beside the road. If this area is somehow full, you can park at the primitive campground.

30

Fort Loudon State Historic Area Hike

SCENERY: ★ ★ ★
TRAIL CONDITION: ★ ★ ★ ★
CHILDREN: ★ ★ ★
DIFFICULTY: ★
SOLITUDE: ★ ★ ★

THIS OAK WAS AROUND BEFORE TENNESSEE BECAME A STATE.

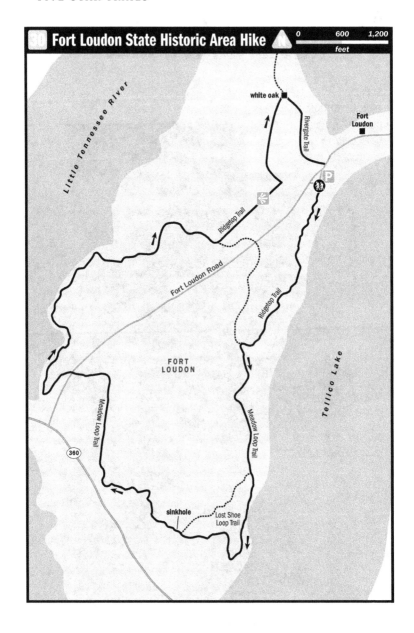

GPS TRAILHEAD COORDINATES: N35° 35.651' W84° 12.510'

DISTANCE & CONFIGURATION: 3.4-mile loop

HIKING TIME: 2 hours

HIGHLIGHTS: Lake views, mountain views, diverse habitats

ELEVATION: 860 feet at trailhead to 950 feet at high point

ACCESS: No fees, permits, or passes required; open 8 a.m.–sunset

MAPS: Fort Loudon SHA Bobby Brewer Trail System, USGS Vonore

FACILITIES: Picnic area, water, restrooms, museum near trailhead

WHEELCHAIR ACCESS: None

CONTACTS: Fort Loudon State Historic Area, 338 Fort Loudoun Rd., Vonore, TN 37885; (423) 884-6217; **tnstateparks.com**

Overview

Make a loop on a water-encircled peninsula at this site of an 18th-century English fort. Leave an attractive picnic area, then travel hilly woods overlooking Tellico Lake. The hike then winds through open meadows before returning waterside. A hill climb leads to rewarding overlooks of the Southern Appalachians. From there, drop to a homesite and massive white oak tree that has to be seen to be believed. Finally, return to the picnic area, where you can incorporate a visit to the park museum/fort into your experience.

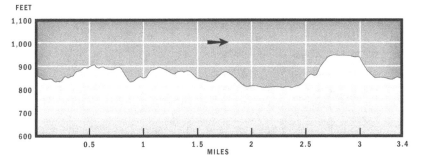

Route Details

Pick up the Ridgetop Trail at the kiosk in the picnic area. Travel south through pine, hickory, oak, and cedar woods on a slope. As you are on a peninsula, Tellico Lake is never far. In this case it is off to your left, easterly through the trees. On a clear day you can easily see the crest of the Appalachians. The natural-surface singletrack path undulates across drainages leading toward the lake.

Bridge ravines at 0.2 miles and 0.3 miles. At 0.5 miles come to a trail junction. Here, Ridgetop Trail heads right, making a shorter circuit. You stay left, now picking up Meadow Loop Trail. Continue traveling through woods, but there is a meadow within sight to your right. At 0.8 miles, you will come to another intersection. Here, stay left with Lost Shoe Loop Trail. It leads left and downhill toward the shoreline. Come directly along the water. The TN 360 bridge comes into view. Climb away from the water, then enter a dense copse of Virginia pines.

Return to meet Meadow Loop Trail at 1.2 miles, still in pines. Interestingly, the trail dips into a wooded sinkhole. Pass above another sinkhole, enjoying a top-down view. At 1.6 miles, the trail opens into a meadow. Rolling hills are covered with tall wavy grasses and sporadic trees. The path is easy to follow, as it is mown through the meadow. Look back to the east as you travel through the meadow for views of the state-line ridge and glimpses of Tellico Lake.

Cross the main park road at 1.9 miles. Reenter woods, heavy with sweetgum trees. Come along the shoreline again, this time on the western side of the peninsula. You're so close to the water that one false step will wet your shoes. Make a northbound track. At 2.4 miles, the path curves abruptly right past an embayment. Begin climbing to the high point of the peninsula and reach a trail junction at 2.8 miles. Rejoin Ridgetop Trail, which really does travel the ridge top here. Wander through a mix of field and trees on an old farm road. Sweeping views of the Smokies and Unicoi Mountains south of the Smokies open up above the fields. What a sight!

At 3 miles, the path reenters woods. Dip to reach a trail junction at an old homesite at 3.2 miles. You can't miss what has to be one of the largest white oak trees in the state. The enormous trunk splits into numerous limbs. Leave right from here, joining Rivergate Trail on a crumbly asphalt road rendered useless by the flooding of Tellico Lake. It is now the final stretch that leads you back to the trailhead.

The English built Fort Loudon here to counter French influence and build relations with the nearby Cherokee during colonial times. Finished in 1756, the fort saw no military action. However, relations between the British and Cherokee turned out badly. The natives laid siege to the fort from March until August of 1760. The British surrendered and left the fort but were attacked and either killed or captured and enslaved. Eventually, many of the survivors were ransomed and returned to their families. The fort was all but forgotten until the early 1900s, when a marker commemorated the site. In 1933, the land was bought by the state and eventually became the preserve we see today. Visit the park museum for a more in-depth Fort Loudon learning experience.

Nearby Attractions

While you are here, consider also visiting the Sequoyah Birthplace Museum, which is just a short distance down TN 360 on your right. Sequoyah, a Cherokee, invented the Cherokee alphabet and developed the written word for the natives.

Directions

From Knoxville, take US 129/Alcoa Highway south through Maryville and join US 411 south of Maryville, heading toward Madisonville. Bridge the impounded Tellico River, coming to Vonore. Look for the intersection with TN 360 at a traffic light. Turn left on TN 360 south and drive 1 mile to Fort Loudon State Historic Area on your left. Turn into the park and follow the main park road 1 mile to a picnic area on your right. Park here. The hike starts at a trailhead kiosk.

Smoky Mountains:
Alum Cave Bluff

SCENERY: ★ ★ ★ ★ ★
TRAIL CONDITION: ★ ★ ★
CHILDREN: ★ ★
DIFFICULTY: ★ ★ ★
SOLITUDE: ★

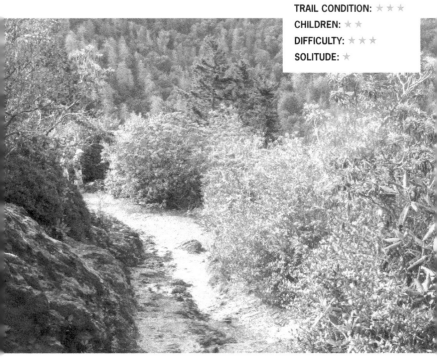

ALUM CAVE BLUFF TRAIL IS BUSY BUT BEAUTIFUL.

GPS TRAILHEAD COORDINATES: N35° 37.690' W83° 27.020'

DISTANCE & CONFIGURATION: 4.6-mile out-and-back

HIKING TIME: 2.6 hours

HIGHLIGHTS: Old-growth trees, great views, natural arch, rock bluff with views

ELEVATION: 3,890 feet at trailhead to 5,000 feet at turnaround point

ACCESS: No fees, permits, or passes required

MAPS: Great Smoky Mountains National Park, USGS Mount LeConte

FACILITIES: None

WHEELCHAIR ACCESS: None

CONTACTS: Great Smoky Mountains National Park, 107 Park Headquarters Rd., Gatlinburg, TN 37738; (865) 436-1200; **nps.gov/grsm**

Overview

Some hikes are busy for a reason, and this one has several, including highlights ranging from spectacular views to old-growth forests to a natural arch—rare for the Smokies—and finally to an overhanging bluff with views of its own. If you time your hike right, you can enjoy these highlights as a less-crowded trek.

Route Details

The steep slopes of Mount LeConte contain some of the most beautiful scenery in the Smokies. The hike travels an ancient forest along Alum Cave Creek before turning up Styx Branch, where Arch Rock awaits. This geological feature is different from the classic arches you may have seen on the Cumberland Plateau; it is more of a circular maw, with stone steps leading through it. The hike then opens onto a heath bald where a rock promontory lives up to its Inspiration Point name. Finally, you climb a rock slope to reach Alum Cave Bluff, a huge rock overhang with views of its own. Try to plan your hike during off times to avoid the crowds. I suggest getting there at sunrise, during times of possible rain, or on winter weekdays. Do not hike here during summer or holiday weekends, as Smokies visitors from afar clog this deserving highlight reel of a hike. It also gets use from folks hiking up and down on overnight trips to Mount LeConte Lodge.

Spur trails from the two large parking areas converge at the bridge over Walker Camp Prong, which you cross by footlog. Old-growth forest of yellow birch and spruce rise above the hiker-only trail as it slices through a rhododendron sea. Bridge Alum Cave Creek on a footlog. Notice some of the hemlocks close to the trailhead are being preserved, but you will also see red spruce, another evergreen. Watch for a massive red spruce to the left of the trail at 0.4 miles. This is a good spot to look around and take inventory of the grove. Authentic old-growth woodland is not an agglomeration of ancient trees. On the contrary, even aged trees are a result of disturbance. An old-growth forest will have many big trees along with younger

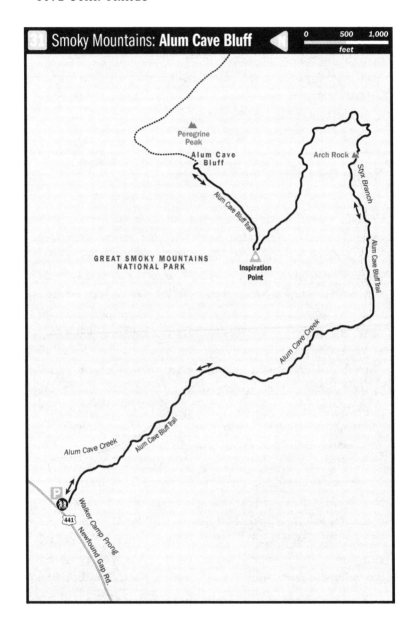

trees that grow when they get the chance. A growth opportunity is created when a big tree falls, creating a light gap. Young trees sprout in this light gap and other already somewhat grown trees thrive in the additional sun. Other times, in the dim of the dark forest, trees gain foothold on nurse logs. Nurse logs are already dead—fallen and decaying—trees that allow a seedling to gain root, then feed the young trees with the energy contained within the decaying log. Later, the new trees grow and spread roots around the fallen log. Over time, the nurse log returns entirely to the soil, and the newly grown tree looks as if it grew up with legs.

The heavily traveled trail is quite rooty, so watch your footing as well as the stately giants above and the crystalline stream beside you, with its beige, gray, and tan rocks. Cross Alum Cave Creek on another footlog at mile 1. The trail swerves left and begins to follow Styx Branch, which it bridges at 1.3 miles. Watch for a gigantic buckeye tree just after this crossing that brings you over to the left-hand bank. Next, come to one of nature's more time-consuming projects, Arch Rock, at 1.4 miles, just after another footlog crossing of Styx Branch. At first, it seems that the path dead-ends. However, a set of stone stairs leads the way through the tunnel-like arch. Continue ascending, stepping over Styx Branch a final time at 1.5 miles. Open onto an area covered with small, low bushes known as a heath bald. Rock outcrops are mixed among the low-slung Catawba

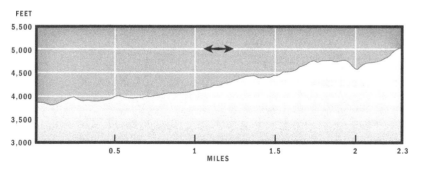

rhododendron, sand myrtle, and mountain laurel, along with a few wind-sculpted trees. Interestingly, sand myrtle grows only along the Southeastern coastline and the Southern Appalachians but isn't found in the hundreds of miles between the distinct ecosystems.

Views open from Inspiration Point at 2 miles, including the Chimneys and Sugarland Mountain across the gulf; the rockslides of Anakeesta Ridge; and slides nearer to the west, where unstable soils have simply sloughed off the mountainside, usually following heavy rain events. Give yourself ample time to relax in this superlative setting.

Leave the bald, cruising the rock face of Peregrine Peak, a stony knob of Mount LeConte. The mostly open rock trail can get quite icy in winter; therefore, the park service has strung wire hand railings along the declivitous slope. Arrive at Alum Cave Bluff, residing at the 5,000-foot elevation, at 2.3 miles. The rock overhang with a dusty floor really isn't a cave. During the Civil War, soldiers led by Thomas Walker and his band of Confederate Cherokees mined the bluff for saltpeter to make gunpowder for the South. You can usually smell the sulfur in the air at the bluff. In winter, large icicles form at the top of the overhang and crash down when the air warms. Nature is constantly at work on the Alum Cave Bluff Trail.

Nearby Attractions

The Sugarlands Visitor Center offers interpretive information, historic displays, restrooms, and water.

Directions

From Gatlinburg, continue south on US 441 to enter Great Smoky Mountains National Park, where US 441 becomes Newfound Gap Road. From the Sugarlands Visitor Center, continue 8.6 miles on Newfound Gap Road to the Alum Cave Bluffs parking area on your left.

32 Smoky Mountains:

Baskins Creek Loop and Spur to Baskins Falls

SCENERY: ★ ★ ★ ★
TRAIL CONDITION: ★ ★ ★ ★
CHILDREN: ★ ★
DIFFICULTY: ★ ★ ★
SOLITUDE: ★ ★ ★

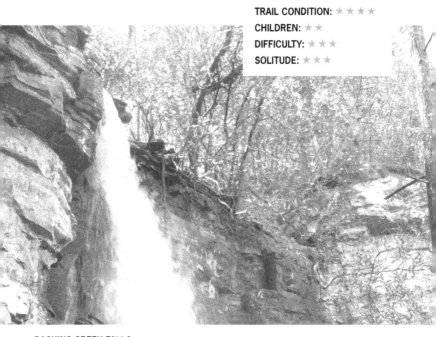

BASKINS CREEK FALLS

GPS TRAILHEAD COORDINATES: N35° 41.720' W83° 28.942'

DISTANCE & CONFIGURATION: 6.4-mile loop

HIKING TIME: 3.7 hours

HIGHLIGHTS: Waterfall, views, homesites

ELEVATION: 2,700 feet at trailhead to 2,110 feet at low point

ACCESS: No fees, permits, or passes required

MAPS: Great Smoky Mountains National Park, USGS Mount LeConte

FACILITIES: None

WHEELCHAIR ACCESS: None

COMMENTS: No pets allowed in park

CONTACTS: Great Smoky Mountains National Park, 107 Park Headquarters Rd., Gatlinburg, TN 37738; (865) 436-1200; **nps.gov/grsm**

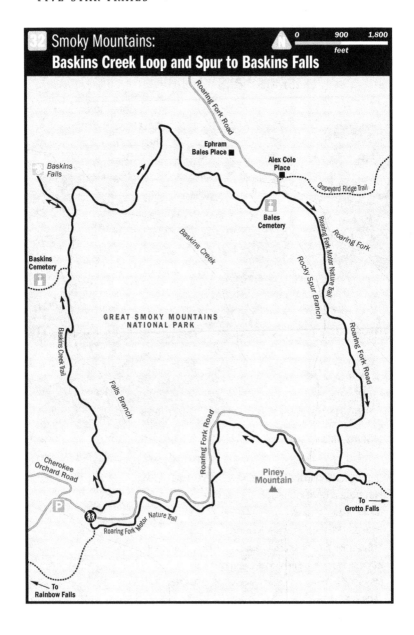

32 Smoky Mountains:
Baskins Creek Loop and Spur to Baskins Falls

0   900   1,800
feet

Roaring Fork Road

Ephram
Bales Place ■

Alex Cole
Place ■

Grapeyard Ridge Trail

Baskins
Falls

Bales
Cemetery

Baskins Creek

Roaring Fork Motor Nature Trail

Roaring Fork

Baskins
Cemetery

Rocky Spur Branch

GREAT SMOKY MOUNTAINS
NATIONAL PARK

Baskins Creek Trail

Roaring Fork Road

Falls Branch

Roaring Fork Road

Cherokee
Orchard Road

Piney
Mountain
▲

To →
Grotto Falls

P

Roaring Fork Motor Nature Trail

← To
Rainbow Falls

Overview

This loop, very near Gatlinburg, travels surprisingly hilly terrain and winds amid multiple ecotones to reach Baskins Falls and some pioneer history. The route then meets Roaring Fork Motor Nature Trail. Hikers walk the motor trail a short way to meet Trillium Gap Trail, which then returns them to the trailhead.

Route Details

Baskins Creek, home to Smoky Mountain pioneers, doesn't seem a likely settler locale; its numerous hills and tight but small valleys challenged those who wished to live here. However, live here they did, in the shadow of Mount LeConte. Now you can get a good workout while seeing a little history, plus Baskins Creek Falls. That cascade is overshadowed by two of the Smokies' better-known cataracts, Rainbow Falls and Grotto Falls, both of which are accessed from this same general area. Avid waterfall enthusiasts could bag all three falls in the same day. Baskins Creek Falls is by far the least visited of them all.

Finding Baskins Creek Trail can be a challenge. It is best accessed where it crosses Roaring Fork Motor Nature Trail 0.2 miles beyond the motor nature trail's beginning, where you should park. Leave left from the motor trail. The hillier-than-you-think path meanders innocently through second-growth woodland before turning uphill

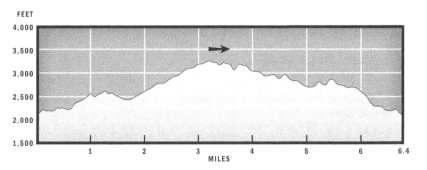

191

onto an unnamed pine, oak, and mountain laurel ridge spurring off Piney Mountain, a shoulder of Mount LeConte. Westerly views of Cove Mountain open. Cruise along this eye-catching ridgeline before steeply dropping to meet Falls Branch, a tributary of Baskins Creek. Step over the stream at 1 mile, soon passing a rock overhang on trail right. Overhangs such as this are uncommon in the Smokies, as opposed to the Cumberland Plateau, west of the Knoxville, where rock shelters and overhangs are ubiquitous.

Just as the hollow of Falls Branch becomes suffocatingly tight, it widens and reveals a sea of rhododendron below, where Falls Branch crashes downstream. Though the falls is obscured by the rhododendron, its watery sounds fill the hollow. The path slips across a small flat to meet a spur trail leading left. This path travels 0.25 miles uphill to Baskins Cemetery, a small pioneer cemetery. All but one grave is unmarked. Baskins Creek Trail continues downstream to meet another spur trail at 1.3 miles. This is the path to Baskins Falls. Trace the quarter-mile spur trail past a pioneer homesite, complete with the broken-down chimney, and down a muddy track. The flat where the homesite stands closes, and the trail drops steeply to Baskins Falls, which spills over a wide rock face in two stages. You will likely be able to enjoy this cataract by yourself, while throngs will be crowding Rainbow Falls and Grotto Falls. Interestingly, pioneers purportedly used Baskins Falls as a natural shower.

Baskins Creek Trail curves over a ridge, then drops to meet Baskins Creek. Step over the stream and meet an old wagon road that goes in both directions along Baskins Creek. Follow the track up Baskins Creek, in another tight hollow made tighter by rhododendron tunneling over the trail. The hollow opens to a final homesite, the highest one on Baskins Creek, before turning up a dry drainage. The subsequent 500-foot climb to the ridge dividing Baskins Creek from Rocky Spur Branch is steep. The trail levels out a bit on the ridgeline, where chestnut oaks thrive, to bisect Rocky Spur Branch. Bales Cemetery is just beyond Rocky Spur Branch on your right and enclosed in a fence. Most of the markers are simple unmarked vertical rock slabs. Meet Roaring Fork Motor Nature Trail at 2.7 miles. The Alex Cole homestead is just down the road and across Roaring Fork.

Now, turn right, heading up Roaring Fork Motor Nature Trail, watching for cars. Also watch for showy orchis and foamflower in spring. Bridge Rocky Spur Branch at 3.2 miles, then come to the well-used connector path leading to Trillium Gap Trail at 3.9 miles. Turn left here and soon reach the actual Trillium Gap Trail. If you want to extend your loop, take a left to Grotto Falls, 1.1 miles distant. The main loop veers right on Trillium Gap Trail. This lesser-used, nearly level path follows an old mountain roadbed, crossing small creeks coming off the side of Mount LeConte. Doghobble, ferns, and rhododendron border the trail as it passes above the Grotto Falls parking area, which has a restroom. Quartz outcrops brighten the woods. Watch for occasional big trees. The path begins a downgrade before it reaches a trail junction near an incredibly gnarled oak tree. It is but a few feet to the right to reach Roaring Fork Road and the end of your loop at 6.4 miles.

Nearby Attractions

Gatlinburg is one of East Tennessee's biggest tourist attractions and offers everything from music shows to off-the-wall museums to anything a tourist will eat.

Directions

From downtown Knoxville take Chapman Highway to Gatlinburg and traffic light #8, Airport Road, 4 miles before reaching the Sugarlands Visitor Center in Great Smoky Mountains National Park. Turn left on Airport Road and follow it 0.6 miles, then keep forward, joining Cherokee Orchard Road to enter the park. At 4 miles, reach the Roaring Fork Motor Nature Trail. Park here. Walk up Roaring Fork Motor Nature Trail 0.2 miles to reach Baskins Creek Trail on your left. In winter Roaring Fork Motor Nature Trail will be gated, but you can simply walk around the gate to access the trail.

33

Smoky Mountains:
Cucumber Gap Loop

SCENERY: ★ ★ ★
TRAIL CONDITION: ★ ★ ★ ★ ★
CHILDREN: ★ ★ ★
DIFFICULTY: ★ ★
SOLITUDE: ★ ★

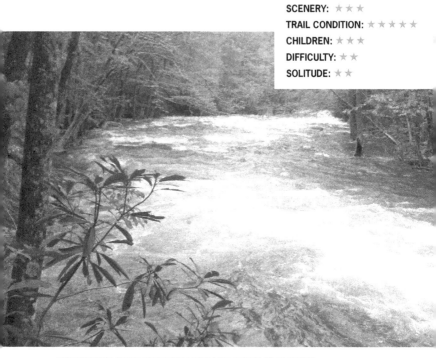

LITTLE RIVER DRAINS THE LOFTIEST TERRAIN IN TENNESSEE.

GPS TRAILHEAD COORDINATES: N35° 39.218' W83° 34.778'

DISTANCE & CONFIGURATION: 5.6-mile loop

HIKING TIME: 3 hours

HIGHLIGHTS: River views, waterfall, national park–level scenery

ELEVATION: 2,200 feet at trailhead to 2,900 feet at high point

ACCESS: No fees, passes, or permits required

MAPS: Great Smoky Mountains Trail Map, USGS Gatlinburg

FACILITIES: Restrooms and water at nearby Elkmont Campground

WHEELCHAIR ACCESS: None

COMMENTS: No pets allowed in national park

CONTACTS: Great Smoky Mountains National Park, 107 Park Headquarters Rd., Gatlinburg, TN 37738; (865) 436-1200; **nps.gov/grsm**

Overview

This is an ideal Smoky Mountains hike for those who want more of a woodland stroll than a lung-busting alpine ascent. Leave the Elkmont area of the park and cruise up the ultra-attractive Little River Valley, where the watercourse tumbles over huge boulders, forming large clear pools that invite a dip in the cool mountain stream. Pass a tributary making a waterfall just as it reaches the Little River. Leave the Little River on an old railroad grade that gently climbs to a gap, then descend to Jakes Creek Valley and return to Elkmont.

Route Details

You'll begin on a path that was part of the Little River Road until a mid-1990s flood washed out this upper section. The park service decided to move the trailhead back rather than repair the road.

Pass through the former Elkmont summer home community, known as the Appalachian Club, on a crumbling asphalt path. Vestiges of the stone entry gates and summer cottages survive. After 0.25 miles, you leave the old summer cottage community on a wide gravel track shaded by tulip trees, sycamore, black birch, yellow birch, and scads of doghobble rhododendron mixed with mossy boulders. The sparkling Little River lies to the left, always trying to lure you to its banks with attractive shoals, crystalline pools, small islands, and big rocks ideal for sunning or feeling the cool breeze flow down the valley. At 0.4 miles, Bearwallow Branch comes in on your right.

At 1 mile, the path narrows after you pass the old parking area. A bluff pinches the trail to the river in places. In other spots the Little River is only audible, not visible. The Little River drains the highest point in the Smokies, Clingmans Dome, then gathers tributaries, flowing north and west through the park before emerging near the community of Townsend. From there it continues northwest to meet the Tennessee River near Maryville.

Burnt Mountain rises to your right, and this hike leads completely around the wooded peak. At 2 miles, Huskey Branch

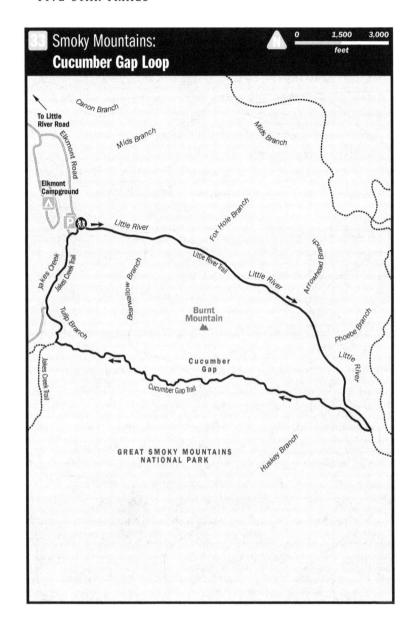

flows beneath a bridge into the Little River and a large pool below. Here, Huskey Branch tumbles as a multitier cascade above and below the trail as it slices through jagged rock. Look into the pool below for swimming trout. Brook trout, technically a char, are the only native trout in the Smokies. However, brown trout and rainbow trout have been introduced into the park and thrive in its waters. In the lower Little River you are most likely to see brown and rainbow trout.

Keep walking for a bit, coming to an intersection with the Cucumber Gap Trail at 2.4 miles. Turn right onto the Cucumber Gap Trail. This path may have more vines among the trees than any other trail in the park. Ascend an old railroad grade, rock-hopping Huskey Branch at mile 2.8. Muscadine vines are prominent elements of the trailside forest. The small native grapes ripen in early fall and are favored by all sorts of wildlife in the Smokies. The thick-skinned fruit grows throughout the Southeast, and early settlers used it to make wine. Today's wine makers purposefully cultivate the varietal. The fruit is also touted as a modern-day health food with antioxidants.

The path keeps rising along a small feeder stream of Huskey Branch, crossing it at 3.2 miles. Occasional views open through the trees to the right. The path passes just above Cucumber Gap at 3.5 miles; you are just below 3,000 feet. The gap was named for the cucumber tree, which is part of the magnolia family. Its green fruit resembles a mini cucumber and will be seen trailside in September.

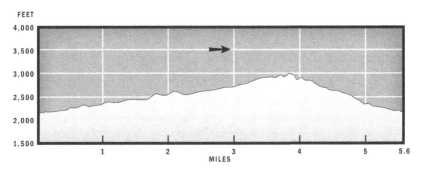

The tree appears throughout the mid-Appalachians, with West Virginia in the heart of its range. Outlier populations stretch to Louisiana and Missouri.

The flat in Cucumber Gap was once home to a Smoky Mountain pioneer family. Look for leveled locations and piled stones in the woods, perhaps reminiscent of those people. Pass some fairly large beech trees and arrow-straight regal tulip trees before descending to cross Tulip Branch at 4.4 miles. Meet the wide Jakes Creek Trail at 4.6 miles. Turn right here and descend to a pole gate at 5 miles. Enter the former summer home community, passing the Jakes Creek trailhead parking area. Keep downhill on an asphalt path open to vehicular traffic to a split in the road at mile 5.5. Turn right here and soon reach the Little River Trail, completing your loop at 5.6 miles.

Nearby Attractions

Elkmont has a large but well-kept and well-loved campground that stretches out just below the trailhead. It offers more than 200 sites and makes a great base camp for exploring the Elkmont area of the park.

Directions

From Knoxville, take Chapman Highway to Gatlinburg and continue into Great Smoky Mountains National Park to reach Sugarland Visitor Center. From here, turn right onto Little River Road and follow it 4.9 miles, then turn left into Elkmont. Follow the paved road 1.3 miles to Elkmont Campground. Turn left just before the campground check-in station and follow this road a short distance to cross the Little River. The Little River Trail starts on the left shortly after the bridge.

34

Smoky Mountains:
Hen Wallow Falls Hike

SCENERY: ★ ★ ★ ★ ★
TRAIL CONDITION: ★ ★
CHILDREN: ★ ★
DIFFICULTY: ★ ★ ★
SOLITUDE: ★ ★ ★

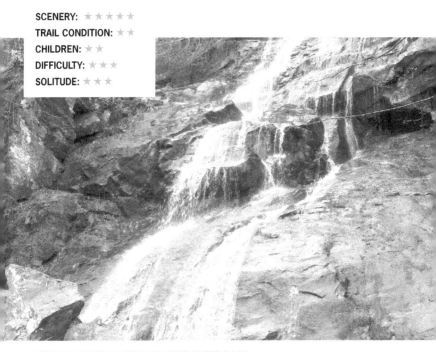

HEN WALLOW FALLS TUMBLES OVER SHEER ROCK.

GPS TRAILHEAD COORDINATES: N35° 45.470' W83° 12.578'

DISTANCE & CONFIGURATION: 4.8-mile out-and-back

HIKING TIME: 2.8 hours

HIGHLIGHTS: Tall waterfall, homesites, mountain streams

ELEVATION: 1,930 feet at trailhead to 3,005 feet at high point

ACCESS: No fees, permits, or passes required

MAPS: Great Smoky Mountains National Park, USGS Hartford

FACILITIES: Picnic area, water fountains, restrooms, campground

WHEELCHAIR ACCESS: None

COMMENTS: No pets allowed in national park

CONTACTS: Great Smoky Mountains National Park, 107 Park Headquarters Rd., Gatlinburg, TN 37738; (865) 436-1200; **nps.gov/grsm**

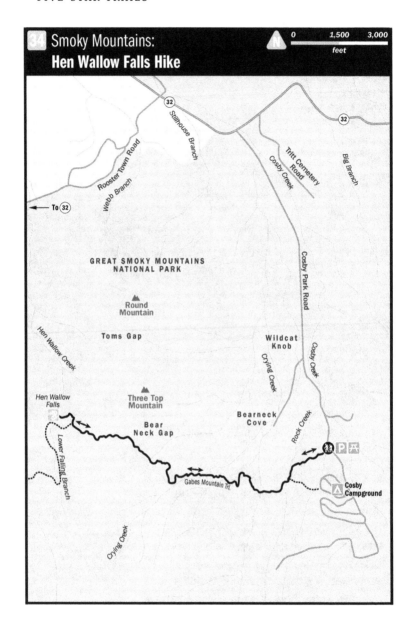

34 Smoky Mountains:
Hen Wallow Falls Hike

0   1,500   3,000
feet

32

Stillhouse Branch

32

Rooster Town Road

Tritt Cemetery Road

Cosby Creek

Big Branch

Webb Branch

To 32

GREAT SMOKY MOUNTAINS
NATIONAL PARK

Round
Mountain

Cosby Park Road

Hen Wallow Creek

Toms Gap

Wildcat
Knob

Crying Creek

Cosby Creek

Three Top
Mountain

Hen Wallow
Falls

Bear
Neck Gap

Bearneck
Cove

Rock Creek

Lower Falling Branch

Gabes Mountain Trl.

Cosby
Campground

Crying Creek

Overview

This hike leaves the Cosby area of the Smokies and travels along several tributaries of Cosby Creek, passing old homesites as it leaves flatter ground for Gabes Mountain. It continues a more-up-than-not trek deeper into the Smokies to reach Bear Neck Gap. The terrain steepens, creating ideal conditions for a precipitous waterfall. Take a spur trail to Hen Wallow Falls, a ribbon of white flowing over a rock face, crashing into a pile of rock, creating a fine, lesser-visited Smokies destination.

Route Details

There are many popular waterfall destinations in the Smokies. Hen Wallow Falls is down on that list. True, it doesn't have the volume and power of Abrams Falls or the remoteness of Ramsey Cascades or the easy access of Indian Creek Falls. Nor does it have the crowds that flock to those cataracts. Rather, Hen Wallow Falls tumbles over a rock face, waiting for visitors. That being said, Hen Wallow Falls has been a destination as long as the Smokies has been a national park. Back in the 1930s, the Civilian Conservation Corps routed a trail from nearby Cosby to the falls, over Gabes Mountain, passing through old-growth forest and on to Maddron Creek and the Maddron Bald Trail. The CCC trail has been rerouted somewhat, but Hen Wallow Falls still waits for visitors.

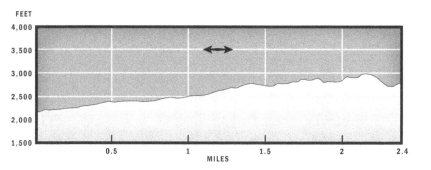

Gabes Mountain Trail begins just downhill from the entrance to the Cosby picnic area. Consider bringing a meal to enjoy here. Cosby also has a large and lesser-used campground that can serve as a fine base camp for the many trails that emanate from the area. Join a rocky track once used by mountain settlers before Great Smoky Mountains National Park came to be. Cosby was one of the most heavily settled areas in the Smokies. A pine-oak-hickory forest shades the trail, bordered by rhododendron and mountain laurel. At 0.1 mile an old road curves left. Stay straight and gently climb to come alongside Rock Creek. True to its name, the stream tumbles noisily down a stony bed. Look down the stream to view smaller warm-up cascades. The trail continues ascending alongside Rock Creek to reach a trail junction at 0.3 miles. Here, a spur trail leads left 0.3 miles to Cosby Campground, allowing campers to access Gabes Mountain Trail directly. Stay right here to bridge Rock Creek on a foot log with a handrail. The bridge allows for unobscured views of the mountain freshet.

The trail narrows as you undulate through rocky woods, stepping over streamlets flowing from Snake Den Mountain. More substantial tributaries have small bridges. Black birch and fading hemlocks grow streamside. Ferns find their place, and moss grows on anything not moving. Bridge Crying Creek before coming to an old auto turnaround at 1.1 miles. In times past this was an auto-accessible trailhead. Pick up a now-narrower trail indicated by a sign, then climb to an old homestead—look for rocks piled in a vain attempt to make this hardscrabble, sloped land more arable. Continue upstream along Crying Creek before turning away at 1.3 miles to shortly pass through an unnamed gap. A little trail leads right from the gap a short distance to a lonesome grave. Here lies Sally Sutton, a Cosby resident. Her grave is marked simply with two stones at either end of the body that lies beneath. Dip to a small stream before rising to reach Bear Neck Gap at 1.7 miles. There's a Smoky Mountains name for you. Rhododendron grows thick on this north-facing spot. The mountain slope sharpens considerably. Vines are draped among the trees of a cove hardwood forest. Pass an open rock face at 2 miles. In wet times water trickles down the face. Winter views open to the north of Three Top Mountain and Round Mountain. More rock bluffs lie ahead.

At 2.2 miles, you'll reach a trail junction. Here, a narrow, rooty track leaves right toward Hen Wallow Falls. Hug a rock face on your descent and shortly you will hear the falls. Reach the cataract at 2.4 miles. A profusion of rocks lies at the base of the 60-or-so-foot falls, which slides in a thin veil over a stone face before splattering into the boulder jumble. Since Lower Falling Branch—the stream that forms the falls—is a low-flow watercourse, consider coming here during winter or spring or after heavy rains. Don't bother with the falls you hear below. The off-trail hiking risk isn't worth the reward. If you want to explore more, continue on Gabes Mountain Trail to see another cascade upstream on Lower Falling Branch and old-growth buckeyes, silverbells, and tulip trees beyond.

Nearby Attractions

Cosby offers a fine campground and trails aplenty for the Smokies enthusiast.

Directions

From Gatlinburg, take US 321 east until it comes to a T intersection with TN 32. Follow TN 32 a little over a mile, turning right into the signed Cosby section of the park. After 1.9 miles up Cosby Road watch for a road splitting left to the picnic area. Turn left here and immediately park. Gabes Mountain Trail starts just a short distance downhill, back toward the entrance to Cosby, on the west side of Cosby Road.

35

Smoky Mountains:
Injun Creek

SCENERY: ★ ★ ★
TRAIL CONDITION: ★ ★ ★
CHILDREN: ★ ★ ★
DIFFICULTY: ★ ★
SOLITUDE: ★ ★ ★

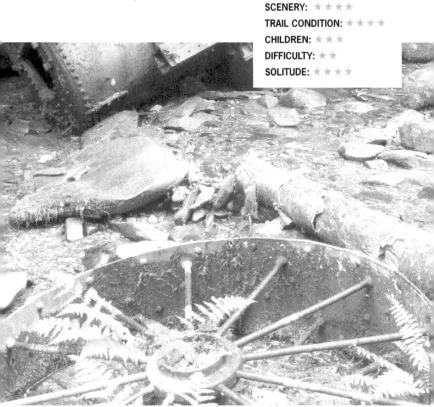

PART OF THE OLD STEAM ENGINE IN INJUN CREEK

GPS TRAILHEAD COORDINATES: N35° 42.510' W83° 22.936'

DISTANCE & CONFIGURATION: 6.6-mile out-and-back

HIKING TIME: 3.8 hours

HIGHLIGHTS: Pioneer relics, solitude, old steam engine

ELEVATION: 1,680 feet at trailhead to 2,580 feet at turnaround point

ACCESS: No fees, permits, or passes required

MAPS: Great Smoky Mountains National Park, USGS Mount LeConte

FACILITIES: Restrooms, picnic area nearby

WHEELCHAIR ACCESS: None

CONTACTS: Great Smoky Mountains National Park, 107 Park Headquarters Rd., Gatlinburg, TN 37738; (865) 436-1200; **nps.gov/grsm**

Overview

Take a walk through time on this secluded hike, which skirts the lower reaches of Mount LeConte, passing a collection of former farms and homesites that dot the Greenbrier area of the Smokies. This underrated and underutilized Smokies trek ends at the Injun Creek backcountry campsite, #32, just above which lies a wrecked steam engine tractor, a high-tech contraption during the pre-park days when it crashed.

Route Details

Greenbrier was one of the most heavily settled areas of what was to become Great Smoky Mountains National Park. Located in the shadow of Mount LeConte, the rocky, mountainous area drains slopes that flow north toward Gatlinburg and Pittman Center. The land is hardly arable, but mountain settlers managed to scrape out a living along the creek bottoms and more sloped tributaries. This hike travels past several homesites located along Rhododendron Creek, a pleasant stream with which you will become very familiar during the several creek crossings the trail makes on its way up to James Gap. From there you descend into the Injun Creek watershed. The old farm–turned–backcountry campsite where you end the trek makes for a great picnic spot. Pull up a rock under the shade of a tree, or simply sprawl out on the grass and contemplate what it might have been like to live here full time without the electrical accoutrements that accompany us in modern life.

Start the Grapeyard Ridge Trail on a Civilian Conservation Corps–built path that cobbles together old roads used by area settlers, passing rock walls and other wagon tracks splintering off the one you're following. At 0.3 miles, on a left-turning switchback, a spur path leads right to a pioneer cemetery. Mixed woodland of

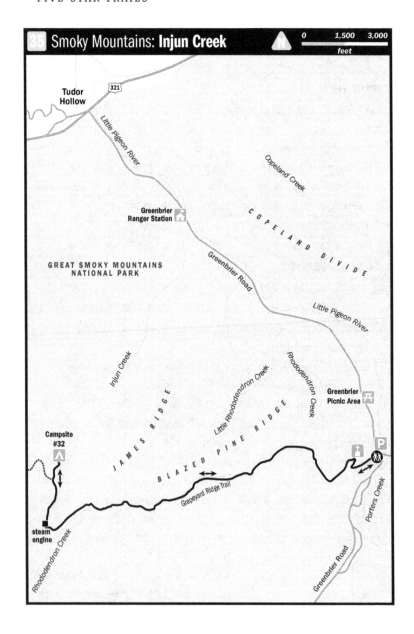

Smoky Mountains: **Injun Creek**

0   1,500   3,000
feet

Tudor
Hollow

321

Little Pigeon River

Copeland Creek

Greenbrier
Ranger Station

C O P E L A N D   D I V I D E

GREAT SMOKY MOUNTAINS
NATIONAL PARK

Greenbrier Road

Little Pigeon River

Injun Creek

Little Rhododendron Creek

Rhododendron Creek

Greenbrier
Picnic Area

J A M E S   R I D G E

B L A Z E D   P I N E   R I D G E

Campsite
#32

Grapeyard Ridge Trail

steam
engine

Rhododendron Creek

Porters Creek

Greenbrier Road

sweetgum, holly, maple, and pine form the forest. Ascend to a gap, on top of which sits an old homesite and the remains of a chimney, at 0.6 miles. The dull roar of the Middle Prong Little Pigeon River fades. The trail follows a small rill leading to Rhododendron Creek in a young spindly forest that was open land fourscore past. At 0.8 miles, step over the small rill and enter a persistent field. Make the first of several crossings of Rhododendron Creek and its tributaries, none of which are deep, though you may wet your shoes a bit in winter or after heavy rains.

Wind up the creek valley, noting homesites on both sides of the path. Watch for exposed trailside white quartz. The 1931 topographic map of the Smokies, commissioned by the Department of the Interior, shows 11 homes in the Rhododendron Creek watershed. Watch for more persistent fields in stream bottoms, which contrast greatly with the numerous rhododendron tunnels through which you pass. At 1.8 miles, a rock marks a spur trail leading left to a confusing network of old roads leading to forgotten homesites and graves of settlers who left the Smokies after it became a park. On down the trail, see where stones line the creek, marking a pioneer's attempt to tame Rhododendron Creek. Farmers knew this rocky land couldn't afford to lose precious topsoil to sporadic flash floods that crashed through the valley.

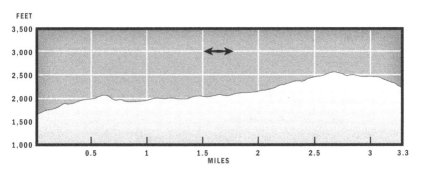

At 2.1 miles, leave Rhododendron Creek and begin the steady ascent to James Gap. A green cornucopia of rhododendron, mountain laurel, moss, and galax flank the path. Oaks and hickories stand overhead and drop their mast on the trail in fall. Another homesite, marked with a mere pile of rock rubble, sits in the saddle of James Gap at 2.8 miles. Enter the Injun Creek watershed. As you descend, the inspiration for the name Injun Creek appears in a rivulet on your right. The body and wheels of a tractor-like steam engine stand upturned, water running beneath them. Somewhere in the naming of this creek an errant mapmaker thought the name Injun Creek referred to the Cherokee that roamed this land long ago and not a steam engine that made its final turn in the Smoky Mountains.

The old road-turned-trail descends to reach the side trail to Injun Creek backcountry campsite #32. Turn right on the side trail to the camp at 3.2 miles and enter yet another homesite. Walk around and look at the lasting changes the settlers made on the land, such as leveling the ground with rock walls. The campsite makes for a good break spot. On your return journey, visualize this area in the future as the forest continues reestablishing its dominion over the Smokies.

Nearby Attractions

The Greenbrier area of the park offers other hiking trails, fishing, swimming, and picnicking.

Directions

From traffic light #3 on US 441 in Gatlinburg, take US 321/East Parkway 6.1 miles to the Greenbrier section of the park. Turn right and drive up Greenbrier Road 3.1 miles to the intersection with Ramsey Prong Road, which crosses a bridge to your left. Park just before the intersection. Grapeyard Ridge Trail starts on the right side of Greenbrier Road.

36 Smoky Mountains:
Little Bottoms Loop

SCENERY: ★ ★ ★ ★ ★
TRAIL CONDITION: ★ ★ ★
CHILDREN: ★ ★
DIFFICULTY: ★ ★ ★ ★
SOLITUDE: ★ ★ ★

GPS TRAILHEAD COORDINATES:
N35° 36.556' W83° 56.115'

DISTANCE & CONFIGURATION:
11.3-mile balloon loop

HIKING TIME: 6 hours

HIGHLIGHTS: Views, Abrams Creek gorge

ELEVATION: 1,100 feet at trailhead to 2,050 feet at high point

ACCESS: No fees, permits, or passes required

MAPS: Great Smoky Mountains National Park, USGS Calderwood, Blockhouse

FACILITIES: Seasonal restrooms, water fountain at Abrams Creek Campground

WHEELCHAIR ACCESS: None

CONTACTS: Great Smoky Mountains National Park, 107 Park Headquarters Rd., Gatlinburg, TN 37738; (865) 436-1200; **nps.gov/grsm**

Overview

This long loop takes place in the Smokies' lesser-visited western lowlands. Leave Abrams Creek Ranger Station on the rolling Cooper Road Trail, passing quiet streams and fire-affected pine-oak woodlands. Join slender Hatcher Mountain Trail to reach the Abrams Creek gorge. Travel past open rock bluffs with views, then hike alongside this gorgeous stream, the Smokies' lowest-elevation waterway.

Route Details

This loop hike is easier than the mileage may indicate. It is every bit of 11.3 miles, and is in the Smokies, but elevation changes are neither long nor drastic. Allow ample time for rest breaks and you can make this a magnificent all-day outing. It is best hiked in fall, when the leaves are changing, but spring and winter are great too. The trail doesn't rise much above 2,000 feet, keeping winter temperatures

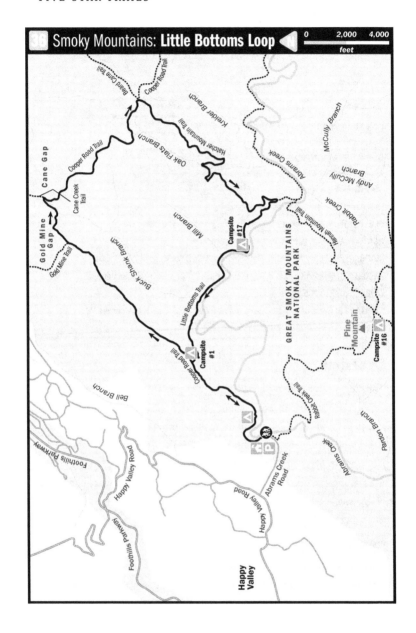

moderate for the Smokies, and in May mountain laurel blooms in the Abrams Creek gorge are a remarkable sight.

Leave the parking area and walk the gravel road upstream along Abrams Creek to reach the end of 16-site Abrams Creek Campground at 0.4 miles. Pass around a pole gate, joining Cooper Road Trail as it traverses a streamside flat with towering white pines overhead. Beech, maple, and holly populate the understory. Rise over a small bluff, then descend to Kingfisher Branch at 0.9 miles. The trail and stream become one for a short distance, then divide.

Reach a trail junction at 1.3 miles. Your return route, Little Bottoms Trail, leaves right. Keep straight on Cooper Road Trail, shortly passing Cooper Road backcountry campsite #1. This former homesite is the lowest-elevation backcountry campsite in the park. It is odd to contemplate, but the rich woods through which you travel were a farmer's cornfield a century back. Continue upstream, stepping over Kingfisher Creek at 1.9 miles. Continue uphill more than not in a white pine–white oak complex. Step over a tributary of Buck Shank Branch at 2.7 miles. Level off in Gold Mine Gap at 3 miles. Stay with Cooper Road Trail as it descends steeply and then levels off to reach another trail junction at 3.4 miles. Here, Cane Gap Trail keeps straight, but Cooper Road Trail, our route, curves right and uphill past Rugel's Rocks, so named for the two massive boulders blocking the path, effectively keeping vehicles from continuing, as

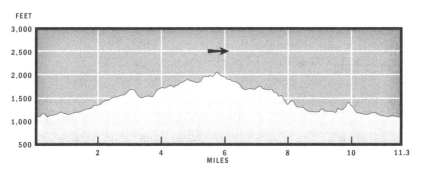

they did in pre-park days. Cooper Road, named for the foreman who built it, was used to connect Cades Cove to the Chilhowee area.

Level off at 4 miles, entering a recovering burn. The scraggly forest may not look so pretty, but periodic fire is necessary to maintain the ecosystem. The fires have also opened more views—at least for the next several years—of Chilhowee Mountain and the tower of Look Rock to the northwest and other ridges to the south. The sandy, gravelly track undulates through more low woods with views, then reaches a four-way trail junction at 5.3 miles. Turn right here, southbound, joining the singletrack Hatcher Mountain Trail. Westerly views open through the pines, maples, and gum trees rising above blueberry bushes. Slip from the east side to the west side of the mountain at 5.7 miles, now going downhill more than not.

At 6.6 miles, step over White Oak Branch in a rhododendron thicket. Soon cross a tributary. Return to dry woods, curving into declivitous Abrams Creek gorge at 7.4 miles. On a clear winter day, Gregory Bald is visible from here. Dip to a hollow full of dwarf irises, then meet Little Bottoms Trail at 7.8 miles. Turn right here, westbound, entering the Abrams Creek gorge. It isn't long before you pass through open rock bluffs bordered by fire-scarred woods. Views open of Look Rock Tower and Chilhowee Mountain, which separates the Smokies from greater Knoxville. The rugged hiker-only path, nicknamed the "Goat Trail," dips to reach the Little Bottoms backcountry campsite #17 spur trail at 8.4 miles, then saddles alongside Abrams Creek. Enjoy close-up stream panoramas, while occasionally climbing mountain laurel–cloaked hillsides. Step over Buck Shank Branch at 9.4 miles, then surmount a low ridge. Cruise through young forest. A pair of switchbacks drops you into thick forest along Kingfisher Creek, and you'll encounter a trail junction at 10 miles. You have now completed the loop portion of the hike. It is an easy 1.3-mile backtrack to the Abrams Creek parking area.

Nearby Attractions

Abrams Creek has an intimate and attractive 16-site primitive campground generally open from March through October. For exact opening and closing dates, check the national park website at **nps.gov/grsm**.

Directions

From Knoxville take US 129 south/Alcoa Highway through Maryville and on to Chilhowee Lake. Once at Chilhowee Lake, continue to the intersection with the Foothills Parkway. From there, keep south on US 129 0.5 miles farther to Happy Valley Road. Turn left on Happy Valley Road, following it 6 miles to Abrams Creek Road. Turn right on Abrams Creek Road and drive 0.7 miles, passing the ranger station. The parking area is on the right just after the ranger station. Cooper Road Trail starts at the rear of the campground. Park your car in the designated area near the ranger station and do not park in the campground, which is gated during the cold season.

37

Smoky Mountains:
Porters Flat Hike

SCENERY: ★ ★ ★ ★
TRAIL CONDITION: ★ ★ ★
CHILDREN: ★ ★ ★
DIFFICULTY: ★ ★
SOLITUDE: ★ ★ ★

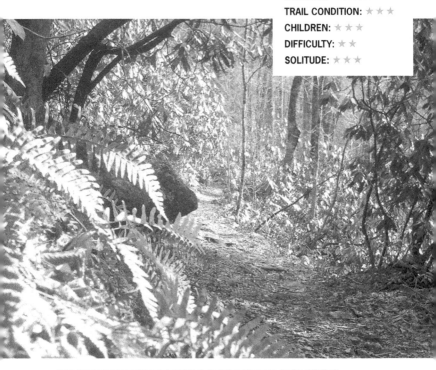

THE SMOKY MOUNTAINS DESERVE THEIR NATIONAL PARK STATUS.

GPS TRAILHEAD COORDINATES: N35° 41.814' W83° 23.272'

DISTANCE & CONFIGURATION: 3.6-mile out-and-back

HIKING TIME: 2 hours

HIGHLIGHTS: Waterfall, preserved hemlock grove, homestead

ELEVATION: 1,950 feet at trailhead to 2,510 feet at turnaround point

ACCESS: No fees, permits, or passes required

MAPS: Great Smoky Mountains National Park, USGS Mount LeConte

FACILITIES: Restrooms, picnic area nearby

WHEELCHAIR ACCESS: None

CONTACTS: Great Smoky Mountains National Park, 107 Park Headquarters Rd., Gatlinburg, TN 37738; (865) 436-1200; **nps.gov/grsm**

Overview

This trek in the Greenbrier area of the Smokies travels along a crystalline mountain stream to reach a preserved hemlock grove. Next, hike to a delicate falls, streaming over a rock face. On your outgoing or return trip, stop by a former farmstead, complete with historic wood structures.

Route Details

This hike offers many highlights that will have you stopping and enjoying them, unable to get up a head of steam if you are hiking purely for exercise. The valley of Porters Creek, through which you will travel, was heavily populated before the Smokies became a park. Even today, hikers will see squared-off flats, stone steps, and more. This hike visits the Ownby Cemetery as well as the Messer Place, a homesite that was early headquarters for the Smoky Mountains Hiking Club. Also, you will view a hemlock grove being preserved by the park. The dark green cathedral stands out among today's saddening skeletal remains of most hemlock trees. Finally, travel farther up Porters Creek to a cascade sometimes known as Fern Branch Falls. The slender, low-flow stream spills over a tall rock slab but will nearly dry in late summer and fall. Speaking of seasons, Porters Creek Valley is one of the Smokies' most bountiful wildflower destinations, so consider hiking here during that time.

Leave the trailhead, passing around a pole gate on a wide gravel track. Straight-trunked tulip trees rise among doghobble, rhododendron, and ferns. Black birch and buckeye thrive in this boulder-strewn area astride Porters Creek. The translucent waters of the braided mountain stream reveal gray and pale rocks. The walking is easy. Potato Ridge rises steeply to your right. Begin looking for pioneer relics. In winter you will more easily see the old rock walls and stone steps—the remains of an East Tennessee way of life long abandoned, such as that seen at 0.6 miles on your right.

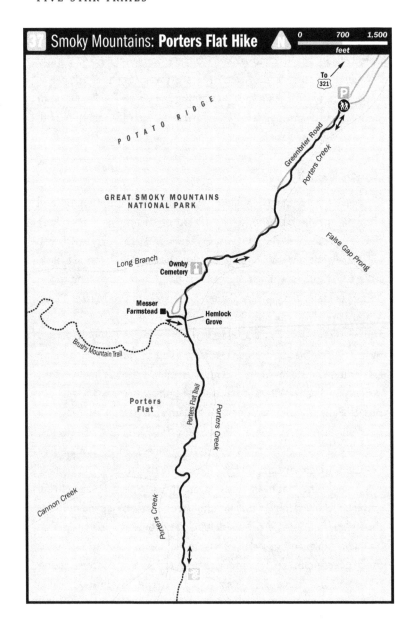

37 Smoky Mountains: **Porters Flat Hike**

0   700   1,500
feet

To
321

P

POTATO RIDGE

Greenbrier Road

Porters Creek

GREAT SMOKY MOUNTAINS
NATIONAL PARK

False Gap Prong

Long Branch

Ownby
Cemetery

Messer
Farmstead

Hemlock
Grove

Brushy Mountain Trail

Porters
Flat

Porters Flat Trail

Porters Creek

Cannon Creek

Porters Creek

Bridge Long Branch at 0.7 miles. Just ahead, the Ownby Cemetery is on your right. You are officially in Porters Flat, a relatively level area surrounded by steep ridges. Pass metal parts of an abandoned jalopy before reaching an old auto turnaround and the preserved hemlock grove. The deep dark greenery was once a common sight in the Smokies, but the hemlock woolly adelgid has devastated the park's estimated 137,000 acres of hemlock woodlands, though so-called "conservation areas" like this one are being preserved by spraying for the pest and releasing beetles that attack the adelgid.

Two trails spur from the hemlock-shaded auto turnaround. Here, Brushy Mountain Trail leads west to Trillium Gap on the shoulder of Mount LeConte, and an unnamed but signed spur trail leads right 200 yards to the old Messer Farmstead. Go ahead and visit the homesite, taking a wide path that curves to a clearing centered with a cantilever barn, a popular style in the pre-park Smokies. Two log cribs hold up the overhanging larger part of the barn. The structure is not entirely original; its wood shingle roof has been replaced along with other elements as needed. Just ahead is the springhouse. Then you reach a homestead occupied by several different owners, the last one being John Messer. These structures were reconfigured into the Smoky Mountains hiking club building we see today. Note the low roof and rock fireplaces.

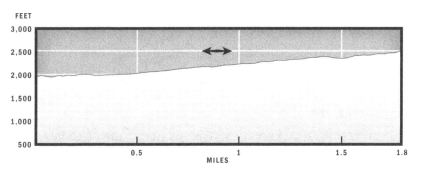

Resume your hike up the now-narrower Porters Flat Trail. Mossy boulders and ferns line the natural-surface track. Bridge Porters Creek at 1.5 miles. Take advantage of this view to absorb the stream scenery, where huge boulders form impediments to frothing water determined to leave its high-country point of origin for Middle Prong Little Pigeon River below.

During spring you have already seen many a wildflower, but beyond here the colorful signs of rebirth reach their densest concentrations. The forest floor is colored with white, purple, yellow, and pink. Old-growth buckeye, white oak, and Carolina silver bell rise among the flower fields. The path narrows and steepens as the northern edge of Porters Mountain rises to your left on the mountainside. In summer stinging nettle will brush against unprotected legs.

At 1.8 miles, look left as a slender falls splashes over an open rock slab to your left. You're more likely to hear it before you see it. The unnamed stream of the falls trickles over the trail. A boulder field stands between you and the cataract, but the falls are easily visible from the trail and make a fitting turnaround point to a great hike. In winter, spring, or after heavy rains, the ribbon of white—Fern Branch Falls—will be more dramatic. If you want to extend your hike, continue 1.4 miles farther to Porters Flat backcountry campsite #31, where the trail dead-ends. Either way, be sure to look for more pioneer evidence on your return trip.

Nearby Attractions

The Greenbrier area of the park offers other hiking trails, fishing, swimming, and picnicking.

Directions

From traffic light #3 on US 441 in Gatlinburg, take US 321/East Parkway 6.1 miles to the Greenbrier section of the park. Turn right and drive up Greenbrier Road 4 miles and park at the end of the dead-end loop.

38

Smoky Mountains:
Rich Mountain Loop

SCENERY: ★ ★ ★ ★
TRAIL CONDITION: ★ ★ ★
CHILDREN: ★
DIFFICULTY: ★ ★ ★ ★
SOLITUDE: ★ ★

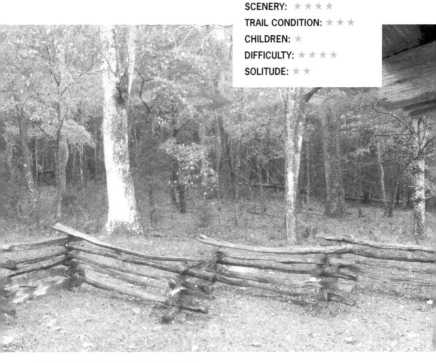

FENCE NEAR THE JOHN OLIVER CABIN

GPS TRAILHEAD COORDINATES: N35° 36.400' W83° 46.655'

DISTANCE & CONFIGURATION: 8.5-mile loop

HIKING TIME: 4.8 hours

HIGHLIGHTS: John Oliver Cabin, multiple views

ELEVATION: 1,940 feet at trailhead to 3,686 feet at high point

ACCESS: No fees, permits, or passes required

MAPS: Great Smoky Mountains National Park, USGS Cades Cove, Kinzel Springs

FACILITIES: Picnic area, campground, water, camp store (seasonal) nearby

WHEELCHAIR ACCESS: None

CONTACTS: Great Smoky Mountains National Park, 107 Park Headquarters Rd., Gatlinburg, TN 37738; (865) 436-1200; **nps.gov/grsm**

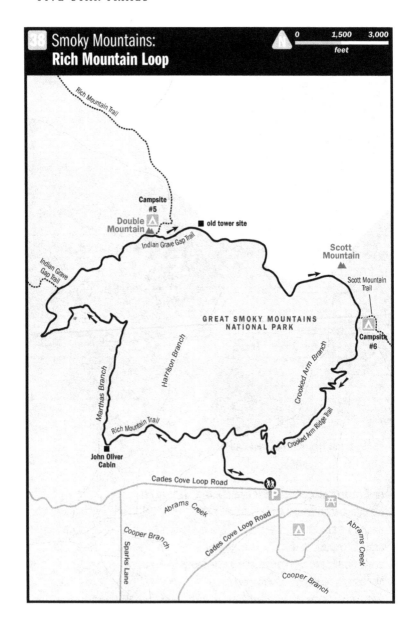

38 Smoky Mountains:
Rich Mountain Loop

Overview

This excellent Smokies day hike shows Cades Cove from a different perspective, a top-down look at the historic farming community nestled against the crest of the mountains. Stop by the historic cabin of Cades Cove resident John Oliver, adding a tangible touch to this exploration of human and natural history of Knoxville's nearby national park.

Route Details

This is perhaps *the* quintessential Smoky Mountain loop hike in Tennessee. It starts in Cades Cove, a point of pride for the Volunteer State. The hike wanders west along the foot of Rich Mountain, tracing pioneer roads with views of Cades Cove. Then the John Oliver Cabin appears at the wood's edge. Walk through pioneer history. The jaunt morphs into an ascent of Rich Mountain. Here, you travel along the a ridgetop and the park border, gaining southward views of the dark, wooded state line ridge across Cades Cove and northward views into Tuckaleechee Cove, toward Knoxville. Visit the former mountaintop tower site at Cerulean Knob, then mostly descend a winding gravelly track with enough switchbacks to make you dizzy.

Start your hike on Rich Mountain Loop Trail, a singletrack dirt-and-rock path. Cades Cove Loop Road is to your left, and Crooked

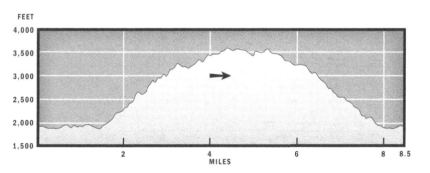

Arm Ridge rises to your right. The nearly level path is shaded by white pines, oaks, and tulip trees. By 0.3 miles, fields open to your left. Gain bucolic views through the trees of waving grasses with wooded mountains beyond. At 0.5 miles, rock-hop over seasonal Crooked Arm Branch, then come to a trail junction. Here, Crooked Arm Ridge Trail, your return route, leaves right. Stay straight with Rich Mountain Loop Trail as it moseys through slightly hilly wooded terrain heavy with shortleaf pines, indicating this was likely pasture or cropland in Cades Cove's heyday a century back. Cross a small, unnamed rocky branch at 0.8 miles as you keep a rolling westerly course amid more pines and sourwood. At 1 mile, step over Harrison Branch. Wander more foothills, then drift into a clearing and the John Oliver Cabin at 1.4 miles. Built in 1820, the cabin serves as a link to East Tennessee's rural past. John Oliver was an early settler of the cove and helped populate it with his many offspring. Other visitors access the cabin from Cades Cove Loop Road.

Leave the cabin and abruptly turn right, up Marthas Branch, northbound on sloping stony land. Note the older trees directly beside the road-turned-trail. The hollow narrows and you pass a crumbled chimney on your right at 1.6 miles. Cross Marthas Branch at 1.7 miles. The trail steepens. At 1.9 miles, the path clambers over an open rock slab. Look at the scratch marks from horseshoes scraping over the rock. At 2 miles, step over Marthas Branch again. Leave the stream for good at 2.2 miles and begin arcing around Cave Ridge, covered in pine and black gum trees. Big boulders appear in the forest. At 2.9 miles, on a switchback, glance down at Cades Cove—the fields seem a lot smaller! You are now at 3,000 feet. At 3.3 miles, meet Indian Grave Gap Trail on the ridgecrest of Rich Mountain.

Join Indian Grave Gap Trail as it gently climbs along Rich Mountain. Gain obscured views across Cades Cove. At 4.2 miles, Rich Mountain Trail leaves left. Backcountry campsite #5 is just down that path. Continue up Indian Grave Gap Trail and enjoy the opening views. Reach a junction at 4.4 miles. Here, a spur trail leads left to the old fire tower atop Cerulean Knob. The four concrete tower supports remain, as does a flat below the knob, with a well or catch basin to serve the tower keeper's cabin once located there. The forest cover limits the views now, but the clearing makes an ideal picnic spot.

Start descending easily along Rich Mountain. Enjoy your hard-earned highland forest cruise. More northward views open into Tuckaleechee Cove. Pass an odd flat that once was a power line pad before meeting Scott Mountain Trail at 5.8 miles. Stay right, joining Crooked Arm Ridge Trail. The path soon divides, then comes back together in a brief confusing section. Switchback down toward Cades Cove. One turn follows another on the rocky path. Some trail users have shortcut the switchbacks. Don't follow their lead, as erosion follows shortcuts.

Step over Crooked Arm Branch at 7.6 miles. Trace the stream downhill on a moderate slope and intersect Rich Mountain Loop Trail at 8 miles. From here, backtrack to reach the trailhead at 8.5 miles.

Nearby Attractions

Bicyclers love to pedal 10-mile Cades Cove Loop Road. The road is closed to vehicles Wednesday and Saturday mornings before 10 a.m. during the warm season, though bicyclists can pedal the road anytime from dawn to dusk.

Directions

From Knoxville, take US 129 south to Maryville and US 321. Follow US 321 to Townsend, Tennessee. At a traffic light, keep straight on TN 73 to enter the park at the "Townsend Wye." Turn right on Laurel Creek Road and follow it 7.4 miles to the beginning of Cades Cove Loop Road. Park at the loop's beginning in the large parking area on the left. To pick up Rich Mountain Loop Trail, walk a short distance down the loop road, past the pole gate; the signed trails begin on your right.

39 **Smoky Mountains:**
Walker Sisters Place via
Little Greenbrier Trail

SCENERY: ★ ★ ★ ★ ★
TRAIL CONDITION: ★ ★ ★
CHILDREN: ★ ★ ★
DIFFICULTY: ★ ★ ★
SOLITUDE: ★ ★ ★

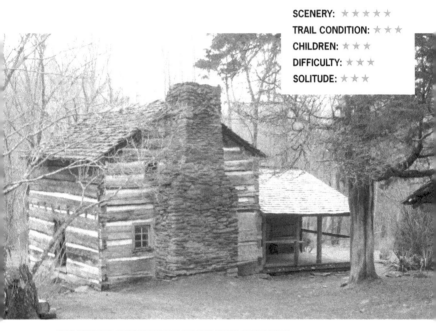

**THE WALKER SISTERS WERE AMONG THE LAST NATIVE
SMOKY MOUNTAIN RESIDENTS.**

GPS TRAILHEAD COORDINATES: N35° 41.678' W83° 38.759'

DISTANCE & CONFIGURATION: 5-mile out-and-back

HIKING TIME: 3 hours

HIGHLIGHTS: Mountain views, historic Smoky Mountain homestead

ELEVATION: 1,890 feet at trailhead to 2,280 at high point

ACCESS: No fees, passes, or permits required

MAPS: Great Smoky Mountains National Park, USGS Wear Cove

FACILITIES: None

WHEELCHAIR ACCESS: None

COMMENTS: No pets allowed in national park

CONTACTS: Great Smoky Mountains National Park, 107 Park Headquarters Rd.,
Gatlinburg, TN 37738; (865) 436-1200; **nps.gov/grsm**

Overview

This scenic ridgeline hike presents views, then visits one of the last working pioneer homesteads in the Smokies. Start at a gap on the Little Greenbrier Trail straddling the national park boundary. The vistas are numerous from a pine-cloaked mountainside before reaching a second gap. Descend a hollow and reach the Walker Sisters Place, occupied by spinster siblings until 1964.

Route Details

This hike travels a ridgeline that seemingly divides time periods in East Tennessee. On one side there is the preserved Smoky Mountains National Park, where the Walker Sisters Cabin—your destination— exemplifies a simpler time, when the Smokies were truly the back of beyond, where homesteaders would spend a lifetime and maybe never even get to Knoxville, much less more distant places. And on the other side of the ridge we see modern "homesteaders" staking out a home in Wears Valley to be near the beauty that is the national park, changing it from a land of the forgotten to an urban outpost. Your mind may contemplate such things as you walk the ridge known as Little Mountain, forming the border of the Smokies.

Begin this hike at Wear Cove Gap on the Little Greenbrier Trail. Climb through archetypal pine-oak–mountain laurel forest on a narrow pathway. Blueberries are abundant in sunnier locales. This path skirts the park border in several places—you will see boundary signs here and there. Also, look down at the elaborate stonework by trail makers that keeps the path from sliding down the mountainside. Views open north beyond the park, especially at a gap at 0.5 miles.

Hike more up than down, then curve around the south side of Little Mountain at 1 mile. Listen for flowing water in the lowlands below. Enjoy good looks into the heart of the park. Numerous dead pine snags are the result of the natural relationship between pines and the native pine beetle. The snags are now falling, and younger trees are taking their place. The walking is easy, allowing you to enjoy

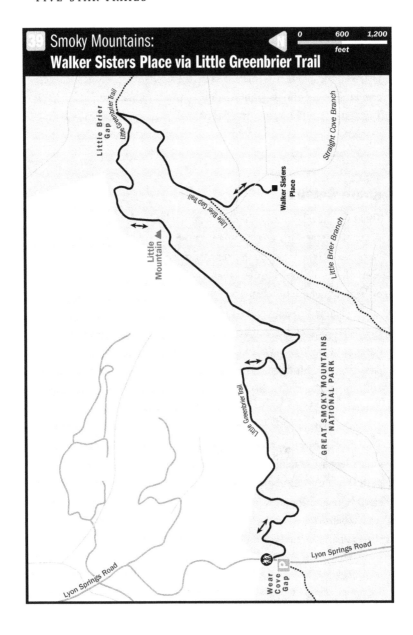

39 Smoky Mountains:
Walker Sisters Place via Little Greenbrier Trail

more views into Wear Cove and Cove Mountain to the east. Descend the ridge of Little Mountain to reach Little Brier Gap and a trail junction at mile 1.9. Turn right here, joining Little Brier Gap Trail, descending into the moist cove of Little Brier Branch, flowing to your left. Tulip trees join the forest.

The V-shaped hollow widens. Little Brier Branch gains flow from tributaries. Reach a signed trail junction at 2.3 miles. Little Brier Gap Trail keeps forward as a gravel road, while a spur track leads left to the Walker Sisters Place. Turn left along tiny Straight Cove Branch. The preponderance of tulip trees and shortleaf pines indicate the area was once cleared. Imagine these trailside flats as fields of corn and other vegetables, perhaps some pasture, back when this was an active homestead.

Come to an open area at 2.5 miles and reach the Walker Sisters Place in a grassy clearing. This cove was occupied for 150 years, with the Walker sisters remaining after the national park was established, thanks to a lifetime lease agreement. After they passed away, the park preserved their homestead. Now, the springhouse, main home, and small barn remain. Notice the notched-log construction of the buildings and the non-native ornamental bushes. Walk inside—the low roof required less construction material and also made the home easier to heat. The white stuff on the walls is old pieces of newspaper that were used to brighten and insulate the cabin. A ladder leads

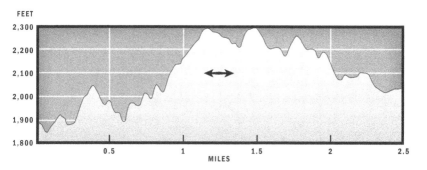

to the sleeping loft. The large fireplace warmed the home, and heat rising up the rock "chimbley" kept loft sleepers a little toastier. The springhouse kept critters from fouling the water and also helped milk and butter stay cool in the summertime. The barn is a smaller version of the cantilever-type barn popular in East Tennessee a century and more ago. Note the farm implements on the wall. If you walk around the perimeter of the yard, you will see other relics, including old car tires that the Walker sisters likely regarded as junk. Remember to leave all artifacts so others can enjoy and discover them. If you are further interested in the area's history, continue down Little Brier Gap Trail 1.1 more miles to the Little Greenbrier Schoolhouse before returning to Wear Cove Gap.

Nearby Attractions

Metcalf Bottoms is 1.3 miles from Wear Cove Gap into the Smokies. It offers picnicking and restrooms alongside Little River.

Directions

From Knoxville, take Alcoa Highway south to Maryville, then join US 321 south toward Smoky Mountains National Park. In Townsend, stay straight, joining TN 73 to soon reach the park entrance at Townsend. Head forward to the "Townsend Wye," a split in the road. Turn left here, onto Little River Road, and follow it 7.8 miles to Metcalf Bottoms Picnic Area. Turn left into Metcalf Bottoms Picnic Area, crossing the Little River on a bridge. Stay on the road for 1.3 miles to the park border, where the Little Greenbrier Trail starts on the right. There is parking here for only one car directly by the trail; another parking area is just over the hill from the trailhead.

Smoky Mountains:
White Oak Sink

SCENERY: ★ ★ ★
TRAIL CONDITION: ★ ★ ★
CHILDREN: ★
DIFFICULTY: ★ ★
SOLITUDE: ★ ★ ★ ★

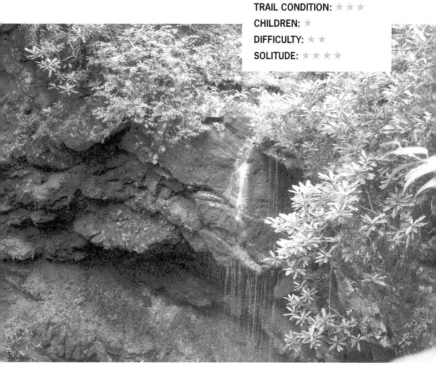

WHITE OAK SINK IS HOME TO AN INTRICATE PLUMBING SYSTEM.

GPS TRAILHEAD COORDINATES: N35° 37.633′ W83° 43.588′

DISTANCE & CONFIGURATION: 4.6-mile out-and-back

HIKING TIME: 2.8 hours

HIGHLIGHTS: Cave, sinkhole, waterfall, spring wildflowers

ELEVATION: 1,650 feet at trailhead to 1,680 feet at turnaround point

ACCESS: No fees, permits, or passes required

MAPS: Great Smoky Mountains National Park, USGS Wear Cove

FACILITIES: None

WHEELCHAIR ACCESS: None

CONTACTS: Great Smoky Mountains National Park, 107 Park Headquarters Rd., Gatlinburg, TN 37738; (865) 436-1200; **nps.gov/grsm**

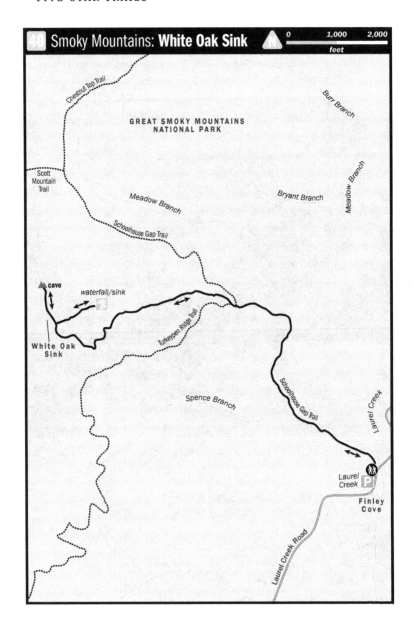

Overview

Take a walk to an off-the-beaten-path Smokies destination—a sink-hole near Cades Cove. Follow an easy track for a little over 1 mile, then dip into White Oak Sink, once home to pioneer families. The sink is also home to some complicated underground plumbing. You can see this manifested in a cave, as well as in a waterfall that drops off a rock face only to disappear into a sink.

Route Details

Even though this Smoky Mountains hike encompasses some hiking on an unmarked trail, the way is clear and the path itself is maintained by the park service, sort of an unadvertised trail. The park service is skittish about too many people coming here because of concerns about rare plants above ground and life in the caves down here. Don't even think about trying to head underground, for your own safety and to allow the belowground habitat to remain undisturbed. You will first follow a historic road built by the first president of nearby Maryville College, Dr. Isaac Anderson. He built the road to connect with settlements over on Hazel Creek in North Carolina in order to share Christianity with them. The road was built only to the state line, then abandoned. Residents of nearby Cades Cove used what became known as Anderson Turnpike to reach the Blount County seat in Maryville.

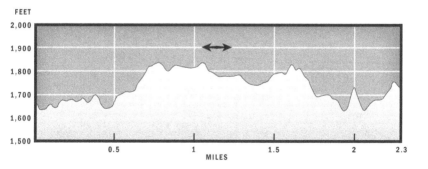

The hike then follows the clear unnamed trail into White Oak Sink. The singletrack path wanders along the slope of a streamlet before dropping off into the flats within White Oak Sink, which is a bowl-like depression encircled by hills. Streams here have no outlet and drain into the ground below. Early residents found the level sink desirable for farming, and several families resided here. Now the sink is left to the flora and fauna, highlighted by impressive spring wildflower displays.

Once in White Oak Sink you can visit two different highlights. First, stop by a cave backed against a rock bluff. A short backtrack will take you to a deep sinkhole into which a waterfall spills, a live demonstration of the intricate underground plumbing in this part of the Smoky Mountains. Just remember to stay on the trail and give this special place the respect it deserves.

Join the wide Schoolhouse Gap Trail as it descends briefly toward Laurel Creek then turns up Spence Branch. Travel directly alongside the small clear stream as it flows over rock slabs in small stairstep cascades. The wide path is shaded by sycamore, witch hazel, and birches. Rhododendron finds its place as the trail heads up a cool, moist hollow, bridging Spence Branch at 0.1 mile. The track suddenly steepens at 0.5 miles, as it heads up a tributary of Spence Branch. Level off in a gap and high point at 0.8 miles. Swing past a persistent clearing on your right. Reach Dorsey Gap and a trail junction at 1.1 miles. Here, Turkeypen Ridge Trail leaves left for Laurel Creek Road, while this hike keeps straight on Schoolhouse Gap Trail. Just ahead, on your left, is the trail to White Oak Sink. The path is clearly visible as it descends left. A stile fence blocks passage by horses and is your "for certain" marker that this is the way to White Oak Sink.

Begin working downhill in a moist valley. Despite not being on maps, the trail is maintained, as evidenced by trailside sawn logs. Come along and cross a small stream in young forest at 1.4 miles. Continue a slim path on a slope. Descend steeply to the sink, entering a flat and rich wildflower area to make a junction at 1.9 miles. Here, trails go left and right. Head left first, walking level ground from which rise regal tulip trees. The trail dead-ends at a gray cliff and cave. The cave is protected by a gate to prevent entry. Other user-created trails explore the flat.

Backtrack to the junction in White Oak Sink. This time take the other path, traveling easterly through more of the hill-guarded plain. Soon the sounds of splashing water drift into your ears, and you reach the waterfall and sink at 2.4 miles. Here, the streamlet you followed into White Oak Sink tumbles over a rock bluff, splashing 30 feet onto rocks and disappearing in a dark, wet maw. In winter, icicles form on the lip of the falls and add frosty splendor to the cataract. Do not walk into the sinkhole. Leave it for the permanent residents of White Oak Sink. From here, backtrack to the trailhead, making sure to stay on the established trails.

Nearby Attractions

Bicyclers love to pedal 10-mile Cades Cove Loop Road. The road is closed to vehicles Wednesday and Saturday mornings before 10 a.m. during the warm season, though bicyclists can pedal the road anytime from dawn to dusk.

Directions

From Knoxville, take US 129 south to Maryville and US 321. Follow US 321 to Townsend, Tennessee. At a traffic light in Townsend, US 321 goes left, but you keep straight on TN 73 to enter the park at the "Townsend Wye." Turn right on Laurel Creek Road and follow it 3.7 miles to the Schoolhouse Gap Trail parking area on your right.

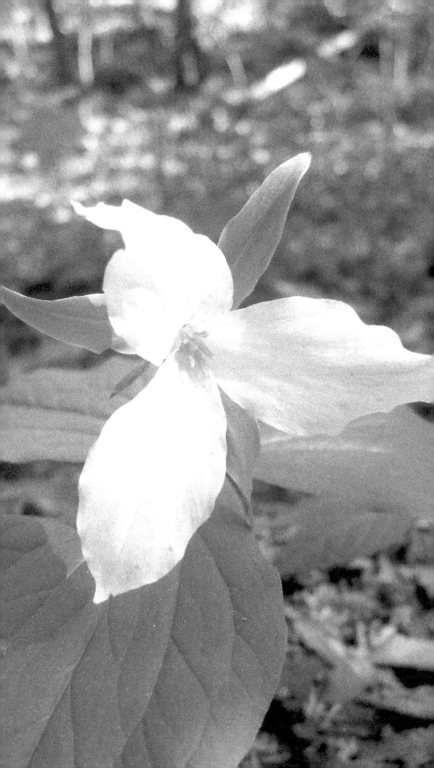

Appendix A: Outdoor Retailers

Following is contact information for outdoors retailers in the Knoxville metro area.

BASS PRO SHOP
3629 Outdoor Sportsman Place
Sevierville, TN 37764
(865) 932-5600
basspro.com

BLUE RIDGE MOUNTAIN SPORTS
11537 Kingston Pike
Knoxville, TN 37922
(865) 675-3010
brms.com

BLUE RIDGE MOUNTAIN SPORTS
4610 Kingston Pike
Knoxville, TN 37919
(865) 588-2638
brms.com

DICKS SPORTING GOODS
221 North Peters Road
Knoxville, TN 37923
(865) 531-2221
dickssportinggoods.com

EARTH TRAVERSE OUTFITTERS
2815 Sutherland Avenue
Knoxville, TN 37919
(865) 524-0000
xgo1.com/ETO

GANDER MOUNTAIN
11502 Parkside Drive
Knoxville, TN 37934
(865) 671-2790
gandermountain.com

LITTLE RIVER TRADING COMPANY
2408 East Lamar Alexander Parkway
Maryville, TN 37804
(865) 681-4181
littlerivertradingco.net

RIVER SPORTS
2918 Sutherland Avenue
Knoxville, TN 37919
(865) 523-0066
riversportsoutfitters.com

UNCLE LEMS MOUNTAIN OUTFITTERS
9715 Kingston Pike
Knoxville TN 37922
(865) 357-8566
unclelems.com

Appendix B: Hiking Clubs

The Knoxville metro area is home to many hiking enthusiasts. Here are some good contacts for clubs and groups that welcome your participation.

SMOKY MOUNTAIN HIKING CLUB
smhclub.org

UNIVERSITY OF TENNESSEE CANOE AND HIKING CLUB
web.utk.edu/~canoehik

GREAT SMOKY MOUNTAINS HIKING AND ADVENTURE GROUP
meetup.com/Great-Smokies-Hiking-Adventure-Group

KNOXVILLE RECREATION AND HIKING MEETUP GROUP
meetup.com/knoxville-adventurers-group/

OUTDOOR ADVENTURE ADDICTS
meetup.com/Outdoor-Adventure-Addicts/

Index

About the Author

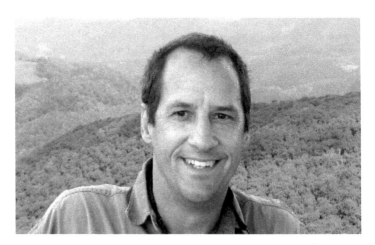

JOHNNY MOLLOY is a writer and adventurer based in East Tennessee, who lived in Knoxville for 20 years. His outdoor passion started on a backpacking trip in Great Smoky Mountains National Park. That first foray unleashed love of the outdoors that has led to his spending countless nights backpacking, canoe camping, and tent camping for the past 25 years. Friends enjoyed his outdoor adventure stories; one even suggested he write a book. He pursued his friend's idea and soon parlayed his love of the outdoors into an occupation. The results of his efforts are more than 40 books. His writings include hiking guidebooks, camping guidebooks, paddling guidebooks, comprehensive guidebooks about specific areas, and true outdoor adventure books. Molloy has also written numerous magazine articles for websites and newspapers. He continues writing and traveling extensively throughout the United States, endeavoring in a variety of outdoor pursuits. His non-outdoor interests include American history and University of Tennessee sports. For the latest on Johnny Molloy, please visit **johnnymolloy.com.**

CPSIA information can be obtained
at www.ICGtesting.com
Printed in the USA
JSHW031007061120
9374JS00012B/200